Common Movement Disorders Pitfalls: Case-Based Learning

Common Movement Disorders Pitfalls: Case-Based Learning

Alberto J. Espay, MD, MSc

Associate Professor of Neurology
Director of Clinical Research
James J. and Joan A. Gardner Family Center for Parkinson's
Disease and Movement Disorders
University of Cincinnati Neuroscience Institute
Cincinnati, Ohio, USA

Anthony E. Lang, OC, MD, FRCPC, FAAN, FCAHS, FRSC.

Professor of Neurology
Director. Division of Neurology
and Jack Clark Chair in Parkinson's Disease Research,
University of Toronto
Director, Edmond J. Safra Program in Parkinson's Disease and
Morton and Gloria Shulman Movement Disorders Clinic,
Toronto Western Hospital
Toronto, Ontario, Canada.

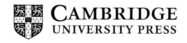
CAMBRIDGE
UNIVERSITY PRESS

CAMBRIDGE UNIVERSITY PRESS
Cambridge, New York, Melbourne, Madrid, Cape Town,
Singapore, São Paulo, Delhi, Tokyo

Cambridge University Press
The Edinburgh Building, Cambridge CB2 8RU, UK

Published in the United States of America
by Cambridge University Press, New York

www.cambridge.org
Information on this title: www.cambridge.org/9780521147965

First published 2012

Printed in the United Kingdom at the University Press, Cambridge

A catalog record for this publication is available from the British Library

Library of Congress Cataloging-in-Publication Data
Espay, Alberto J.
Common movement disorders pitfalls: case-based learning / Alberto J. Espay, Anthony E. Lang.
    p.   cm.
  Includes bibliographical references and index.
  ISBN 978-0-521-14796-5 (Paperback)
  1. Movement disorders–Case studies.   I. Lang, Anthony E.   II. Title.
  RC376.5.E87 2012
  616.8′3–dc23
                                                              2011033927

ISBN 978-0-521-14796-5 Paperback

To our patients, our greatest source of wisdom

Contents

Acknowledgements

The authors thank Drs. Andrew Duker, Francesca Morgante, Don Gilbert, Ruth Walker, Leo Verhagen, Cindy Zadikoff, Héctor González Usigli, Alok Sahay, Alexander Lehn, and Shawn Smyth for sharing some of their cases, highlighting the pitfalls discussed in this book. We are also grateful to Nick Dunton, Senior Commissioning Editor, and Jane Seakins, Assistant Editor in Medicine, both at Cambridge University Press, for their encouragement and professionalism.

Preface

An expert is a person who has made all the mistakes that can be made in a very narrow field

Niels Bohr

Movement Disorders is one of the areas of medicine most dependent on visual observation of patients. Such observation can be subject to many pitfalls. This book has grouped these pitfalls into a catalog of examination oversights, diagnostic errors, and therapeutic disappointments. In this "confessional" of sorts, the reader will appreciate the influence of many case-based educational sessions uncovering diagnoses missed or wrongly attributed, movements difficult to characterize, tests inappropriately ordered or interpreted, and treatments incorrectly chosen or dosed. The wisdom of hindsight thus generated became powerful and enduring lessons that will hopefully leave similarly indelible marks in our readers' medial temporal lobes and limbic system.

The junior author remembers the day when his knowledge on "vascular parkinsonism," hitherto held with scant evidence as rock solid, crashed and burned. Nothing else, in his mind, could have explained the step-wise decline in gait and cognition of an elderly man plagued by multiple vascular risk factors and 60 pack-years of accumulated smoking history. Within this referential frame, an enlarged ventricular system could have only resulted from parenchymal atrophy due to micro-angiopathic brain damage, as the fireworks festering beyond the ependymal fence were then interpreted. Nonetheless, the response to a cerebrospinal fluid diversion procedure, under-taken largely to appease his family, was humbling. This carefully documented outcome, followed by the privileged access to eventual studies on autopsy material, became one among the many powerful lessons that populate the pages of this case-based book.

Organized in nine chapters according to the selected categories of errors and oversights, each case conveys a specific set of clinical pearls on diagnostic or therapeutic issues. It follows in the footsteps of Valerie Purvin and Aki Kawasaki's trail-blazing "*Common Neuro-ophthalmic Pitfalls*" (Cambridge University Press, 2009). With their kind permission and encouragement from Nick Dunton at Cambridge University Press we aimed at mustering a similar coaching style, buttressed by the unique pedagogic wisdom of learning from hindsight. The "hard questions" after each case are meant to steer the discussion straight into the pitfalls – and how they could have been avoided. As with Purvin and Kawasaki's *Pitfalls*, the authors have assumed the readers have a working know-ledge of examination techniques, movement dis-order phenomenology, and neuroanatomic and pathophysiologic correlates of relevant disorders. The cases have been arbitrarily chosen to highlight important weaknesses in the various steps related to the assessment and management of movement disorder patients rather than to represent a comprehensive clinical landscape of the whole of the field. Video segments, in many cases obtained at the initial visit (when a misjudgment may have been committed) and in follow-up (when a diagnostic or therapeutic revision took place), are important com-plementary data, critical to a field so intimately dependent on phenomenological clues.

When the same or related disorder is brought up in different chapters, care has been taken to refer the reader to these complementary sections to enhance the reading experience. For instance, diffi-culties in the recognition of multiple system atro-phy may come from neglecting helpful clinical signs or from missing neuroimaging clues, pitfalls addressed in different chapters. Notwithstanding any overzealous cross-referencing, this book is meant to be read in any order and at any pace. Each individually wrapped clinical sampler stands on its own legs and will hopefully stimulate a range of palatal interests.

The authors hope the reading of the following cases will ease the ride to *Expertise*, that sovereign palace looming on the horizon, tantalizingly within reach after continuously driving the winding and narrow mistake-mined thoroughfare of clinical practice, as it might have been depicted by a Niels Bohr outfitted with a hammer and tuning fork.

Alberto J. Espay
Anthony E. Lang

Diseases discussed in this book

(Spoiler alert: Only browse through this list to stimulate your salivary glands; the thunder of the diagnostic and treatment pitfalls may otherwise be stolen.)

Missing the diagnosis altogether

Case 1: Bizarre ataxia of rapid onset

Case: This 33-year-old woman was admitted to the psychiatry ward, brought by her husband, after rapidly developing a "little girl" speech and inability to remember where she was or what she needed to do. Prior to this admission, she had spent approximately 3 weeks with intractable vomiting, which was reportedly triggered by her remorseful confession to her husband of an extramarital affair. A neurology consultation was called for what were reported as convulsive-type movements in the arms and head, screaming episodes, and a bizarre gait. She had no memory of any of the symptoms forcing her hospital admission. She also complained of feeling that "the ground is moving." The consulting neurologist was informed of a strong suspicion for a psychogenic nature of these patient's symptoms and deficits. A brief examination at the bedside sufficed to endorse the psychiatry team's impression of a psychogenic disorder.

What important piece of historical information was missing in this case?

Her statement of "the ground moving" demanded further attention and should have questioned a psychogenic disorder. At a neurological consultation 6 weeks after her hospital discharge, she described it as the perception of objects around her moving up and down and, also, sideways. This illusory movement of the environment, typically due to the presence of nystagmus, is referred to as *oscillopsia*. A careful oculomotor exam had not been performed. In addition, the history of protracted vomiting prior to behavioral abnormalities should have brought to mind nutritional disorders which may induce oculomotor abnormalities, particularly thiamine (B_1) deficiency.

What element of the neurological examination would support the diagnosis and how to confirm it?

The oculomotor examination is critical in this case. She exhibited upbeat nystagmus, worse on primary gaze (Video 1). Her gait was wide-based and unsteady, and she resorted to a walker for most of her ambulation. Put together, the rapid development of ataxia and nystagmus in the setting of anterograde amnesia should have suggested the diagnosis of Wernicke's encephalopathy, a nutritional deficiency of thiamine brought up by protracted vomiting. Upbeat nystagmus is uncommon and has a relatively short differential list, which includes Wernicke's encephalopathy and paramedian lesions in the medulla and, less commonly, pons and midbrain. The upbeat nystagmus of Wernicke's encephalopathy should be present in primary position (not just evoked exclusively on upgaze) and may be suppressed or converted to downbeat nystagmus on convergence. Other obvious oculomotor deficits reported in Wernicke's encephalopathy are limitation of gaze in all directions and ptosis,

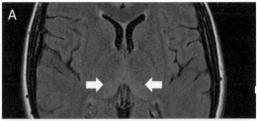

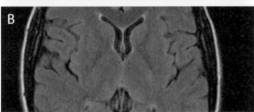

Figure 1.1. Axial FLAIR brain MRI demonstrating mild increased signal in the medial thalamic region when the patient was admitted to the psychiatry unit (A) with resolution after parenteral thiamine replacement 6 weeks later (B). The mamillary bodies, dorsal midbrain, and periaqueductal region, which are other potential targets in Wernicke's encephalopathy, were normal.

which were absent in this patient. The brain MRI from her admission to the psychiatry ward was more carefully reviewed and demonstrated mild symmetric signal increase in the medial thalamus, which had been missed (Figure 1.1A). Thiamine replacement was initiated first intravenously (500 mg) followed by oral supplementation. The oscillopsia disappeared and the abnormal signal intensity on MRI resolved (Figure 1.1B), though her gait did not return to baseline, possibly due to the delay in initiation of therapy.

What other condition should have been suspected in this setting?

With a prodrome of intractable vomiting, followed by ataxia, cognitive or behavioral deficits, and upbeat nystagmus in a young woman having recently confessed to an affair, arsenic poisoning could have also been suspected. Arsenic poisoning is in the short differential list of conditions potentially presenting with upbeat nystagmus and a picture of Wernicke's encephalopathy. Sampling of hair and nails would have been an important screening test while she was in the psychiatry ward, at a time when a putative arsenic exposure would have been recent enough to remain detectable.

Discussion: The sudden onset of an amnestic syndrome complicated by truncal ataxia and upbeat nystagmus following a 3-week period of vomiting should have alerted the consulting neurologist as to the presence of Wernicke's encephalopathy from hyperemesis-induced thiamine deficiency. This disorder typically arises as a result of thiamine deficiency in patients with chronic alcoholism, hyperemesis gravidarum, anorexia nervosa, renal insufficiency, or after the effects of prolonged starvation or IV therapy, and subtotal gastrectomy. The latter may be missed if patients are embarrassed to acknowledge this aspect of their medical history. Also there may be atypical symptoms such as optic neuropathy, papilledema, deafness, seizures, asterixis, weakness, or sensory and motor neuropathy developing as late as 18 months after bariatric surgery complicated with thiamine deficiency.[1] The full triad of eye signs (nystagmus with or without ophthalmoplegia and ptosis), global confusion, and ataxia of gait is seen only in a minority of patients. Pathology shows symmetric demyelination, petechial hemorrhages, and gliosis of midline gray matter areas, such as the cerebral aqueduct, and areas surrounding the third and fourth ventricles. The mammillary bodies are affected in 75% of cases, and the dorsomedial thalamus, hypothalamus, vestibular nuclei, and superior cerebellar vermis in just over 50%. Hence, a normal brain MRI should not detract from initiating thiamine in someone with an otherwise suggestive clinical picture.

In the setting of an abrupt onset such as in this patient, particularly with her "confusional state" and symmetric lesions in the paramedian thalamus, a top-of-the-basilar syndrome due to occlusion of posterior thalamoperforating arteries could be suspected.

Only a minority of cases diagnosed at autopsy (20%) present with the full clinical triad and MRI findings, and many (approximately 30%) exhibit only mental changes.[2] The diagnosis of Wernicke's encephalopathy rests on the recognition of the clinical picture and response to thiamine. Measurement of blood thiamine levels by high performance liquid chromatography, erythrocyte transketolase activity (a B_1-dependent enzyme), or pyruvic acid (B_1 is an essential cofactor for the mitochondrial enzymes pyruvate dehydrogenase and α-ketoglutarate dehydrogenase) can be used to confirm thiamine deficiency.

Established or presumptive Wernicke's encephalopathy is treated with high-potency vitamin B complex. This includes a minimum of thiamine 100 mg IV for 3 days followed by daily B complex with thiamine 250 mg for 5 days or until clinical improvement ceases. Parenteral thiamine replacement improves ocular abnormalities within hours to a few days whereas confusion and ataxia have slower improvement rates. The amnestic syndrome may not recover in roughly 25% of patients, with higher rates when treatment is delayed.

Diagnosis: Wernicke encephalopathy

Tip: *Sudden onset of "bizarre" gaits and abnormal behaviors do not necessarily mean a psychogenic disorder. A full oculomotor exam of an ataxic and amnestic patient would have revealed the diagnosis and avoided delayed thiamine replacement. Paramedian gray matter lesions, even if suspected to represent a stroke, warrant an empiric trial with thiamine.*

Case 2: Staggering progression of gait impairment, urinary incontinence, and dementia

Case: This 80-year-old man with a 60 pack-year smoking habit, hypertension, and hypercholesterolemia presented with a 30-month history of step-wise progression of gait impairment, balance impairment, and memory loss. He had experienced multiple falls and two hospitalizations for sudden-onset freezing of gait. Over the 9 months before presentation, he had become incontinent of urine. His short-term memory had progressively worsened for the past few years. L-dopa, increased to a dose of 600 mg/day, had failed to alleviate his symptoms. The patient resided in a rehabilitation facility where he received assistance with gait and transfers but he was able to bathe, dress, and feed without assistance. His past medical history was positive for hypertension, hypercholesterolemia, and microangiopathic brain disease. He had accumulated a 60 pack-year smoking habit, though he had stopped smoking 40 years before presentation.

What diagnosis reflexively sprang to mind to the examiner upon getting this story?

The step-wise rather than gradual progression along with a couple of stroke-like events in the form of sudden-onset gait impairment occurring in someone with vascular risk factors and heavy smoking history suggested vascular parkinsonism (VaP).

Indeed, the examination that followed did not deter the clinician from this diagnosis. Although his Mini-Mental State Examination score was 25 out of 30, over the course of 2 years, his Mattis Dementia Rating Scale-2 score went from 137 to 92 (abnormal <124) and his Frontal Assessment Battery from 17 out of 18 to 8 (abnormal <13). He had snout and palmomental reflexes. He exhibited a short-stride gait without stooping, shuffling, or festination (Video 2a). He had mild paratonia in the upper limbs but no rigidity in the legs or neck. There was mild hypesthesia to temperature and light touch in a stocking-glove distribution. His postural reflexes were impaired.

Did the brain MRI support the working diagnosis of vascular parkinsonism?

Yes – or so the evaluating clinician suspected. The images were interpreted as representing moderate periventricular small-vessel ischemic disease with

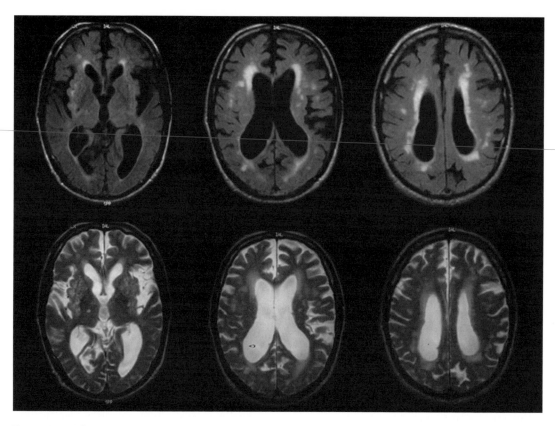

Figure 1.2. Axial FLAIR (upper row) and T2-weighted (lower row) brain MRI shows increased periventricular and subcortical white matter signal interpreted as suggestive of small-vessel ischemic disease. Mild ventricular dilatation appears roughly proportionate to the apparent degree of cortical atrophy.

mild associated ventricular enlargement, proportionate to the degree of atrophy. These findings were supportive of the clinical diagnosis of VaP (Figure 1.2).

What is missing in this story?

A dose of humility and skepticism.[3] The family of this patient relayed his family physician's firm diagnosis of normal pressure hydrocephalus (NPH). The neurologist argued that neither the story nor the MRI findings supported NPH and that this was a "slam dunk" case of VaP. However, the family insisted that they wanted to move forward with treatment for presumed NPH. The

neurologist reluctantly agreed to bring the patient into the hospital for a 3-day external lumbar drainage (ELD) procedure, if only to confirm that there would be no response to cerebrospinal fluid diversion and, therefore, no benefit with a ventriculoperitoneal shunt placement.

In response to the ELD procedure the patient demonstrated substantial improvements in gait velocity (>40% straight walk, >200% in turns) and stride length, and modest improvements in cadence (Video 2b). Cognitive parameters also improved over the pre-ELD measurements. On the basis of these data, the humbled neurologist agreed to the family's request for a ventriculoperitoneal shunt (VPS) placement. However, the patient

Table 1.1. Features of gait in NPH/VaP vs. Parkinson's disease

	NPH (and VaP)	Parkinson's disease
Base	Wide	Narrow
Arm swinging	Normal	Reduced
Sensory cues	No effect	Improve gait
Festination	Rare at any stage	Classic when advanced
Response to L-dopa	Typically nil	Typically marked

succumbed to complications related to a bowel perforation from the peritoneal end of the shunt. An autopsy failed to identify any evidence of vasculopathy, instead uncovering the classical neuropathology of NPH (communicating hydrocephalus with leptomeningeal fibrosis and superficial gliosis of cerebral cortex).

Discussion: In reviewing the clinical features on videotape, it is important to note that this patient exhibited the characteristic signs reported in a classic paper by Thompson and Marsden on Binswanger's disease (defined by head CT without post-mortem confirmation). The most important two signs are (1) a relatively more upright posture and better arm swing that could have been expected for the degree of shortened stride length, and (2) the lack of festination, which is the hastening of cadence at the expense of progressively shortening stride length. Festination of gait is typically seen in Parkinson's disease but rarely if ever in vascular parkinsonism, and, as this patient demonstrated, the other important cause of "lower body" parkinsonism, NPH (Table 1.1) (Video 2c).

As for the brain MRI interpretation and the implications for patient care, there were two important pitfalls in this case. First, the periventricular/deep white matter hyperintensities were readily equated to small-vessel ischemic disease by the neuroradiologist and endorsed as such by the neurologist, who adamantly believed the step-wise progression

of deficits in a man with multiple vascular risk factors and episodes of sudden-onset gait freezing could only represent vascular parkinsonism and dementia. It is worth pointing out that the correlation between brain MRI T2-weighted hyperintensities and vascular disease is tenuous and not supported by clinic-pathologic correlations. In fact, post-mortem MRI-pathologic correlations of asymptomatic individuals have shown that periventricular hyperintensities may be associated with myelin pallor, dilatation of perivascular spaces, increased extracellular spaces, and discontinuity of the ependymal lining and subependymal gliosis,[4] opposite to our knee-jerk interpretation of these lesions as indicative of microangiopathy. It is of interest to remember that striatal infarcts are rarely followed by clinical parkinsonism[5] and that clinically normal individuals may have extensive basal ganglia imaging abnormalities.[6] Also, a response to fluid diversion that is necessary for the diagnosis of NPH has been documented in cases of MRI-defined vascular parkinsonism,[7] suggesting that a substantial burden of hyperintense lesions on T2-weighted MRI or FLAIR suggestive of microangiopathy may not be at odds with the operational definition of NPH. The second pitfall is that when any degree of cortical atrophy was suspected, one should ensure that a similar extent of sulci widening is also present in the brain apex to truly rule out an ex-vacuo form of hydrocephalus. In fact, when reviewing this patient's brain apical cuts in detail, the gyri appeared tight without any sulcal widening suggestive of atrophy (Figure 1.3). The lack of true atrophy in this case was supported by a brain weight confirmed to be a healthy 1400 mg at autopsy.

Diagnosis: Normal pressure hydrocephalus

Tip: *Brain MRI interpretation of "small-vessel disease" and ventriculomegaly is fraught with inaccuracies. Hyperintensities do not necessarily imply vasculopathy. Enlarged sulci with entrapped CSF may give rise to a pseudoatrophic pattern in the brain MRI of patients with NPH. Check the apical cuts when in doubt. Finally, various degrees of ventriculomegaly and abnormal white matter signal*

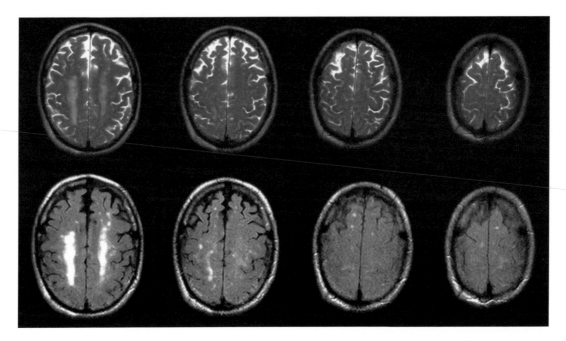

Figure 1.3. Axial FLAIR (upper row) and T2-weighted (lower row) brain MRI of the apical sections of the same patient, showing packed gyri with minimal sulcation suggesting an upward pressure of the brain by the hydrocephalus. At this level, there is no imaging support for the suspected atrophy suggested by the review of the lower-level axial images.

coexist rendering VaP and NPH on a clinical and neuroimaging continuum. Hence, one must be humble about the diagnostic uncertainty and have a low yield to offer lumbar drainage to anyone with a history and examination reasonable for NPH. On the other hand, the patient's outcome emphasizes the need to rigorously evaluate the potential for response to shunting before undertaking this invasive and potentially complicated treatment.

Case 3: Excessive rigidity… and other features

Case: A 55-year-old woman developed very slow gait and progressive stiffening evolving over the 16 months prior to her evaluation. Her husband, a physician, noted a wooden and upright posture with poor flexibility, very short steps, and no arm swinging, reportedly affecting both sides equally.

She developed small handwriting and ultimately inability to grab the pen with her fingers, forcing her to give up writing altogether. She complained of inability to lift the arms above the shoulders. She also noted occasionally blurry vision, slurred and slow speech, and excessive drooling in the evenings, as well as urinary urgency, frequency and occasional mild overflow incontinence. Treatment with low-dose clonazepam had improved the neck stiffness.

Examination showed axial-predominant rigidity with larger limitation in range of motion of passive compared to volitional movements, hyperreflexia, and easy elicitation of what were interpreted as leg spasms (Video 3a). There were no oculomotor or postural impairments. These features were interpreted as highly suggestive of the stiff-person syndrome (SPS). Anti-GAD antibodies were requested and the dose of clonazepam was increased sequentially to a target of 1 mg four times a day.

What features were overlooked?

The greater slowness and amplitude decrement of finger tapping on the left and the reduction in ipsilateral arm swinging while walking were important features overlooked in the early assessment. Indeed, upon re-evaluation 3 months later, she was experiencing excessive daytime sleepiness with the increased dose of clonazepam and acknowledged that her left side was more affected than the right. This brachial asymmetry, which was present early on, had been overlooked in favor of the more striking cervical rigidity. This latter feature, and the reported early response to clonazepam, dominated the early clinical rationale for SPS at the expense of other features that strongly argued against it, such as lack of hyperlordosis and normal range of truncal flexion. The patient was then given a trial of L-dopa and had a marked response at the initial dose of 100 mg three times a day, with normalization of handwriting and substantial reduction of the rigidity (Video 3b). Over the subsequent 4 years she has retained an excellent motor response with an overall increase to 150 mg four times a day, while developing non-troublesome peak-dose dyskinesias and wearing off.

Discussion: When the word "stiffness" is volunteered by a patient with an akinetic-rigid phenotype affecting the range of movement of axial muscle groups, it may be easier to argue in favor of SPS and neglect the more common postural instability-gait disorder phenotype of Parkinson's disease.[8] This diagnostic pitfall resulted from two shortcuts in reasoning: the "framing effect," being swayed by certain aspects of the case more than others; and a "representativeness heuristic," that is, ignoring prior probabilities and base rate frequencies of the different clinical findings. The clinician thought about a zebra (SPS) when hearing a horse's hoof beats (PD). Of course, the axial involvement in SPS is typically lumbar rather than cervical and is often associated with lumbar lordosis. Along these lines, the discrepancy between the voluntary and passive range of motion was not properly interpreted. This patient exhibited clear difficulty with passive rotation of the head in all directions, yet the patient could voluntarily move her head to the extreme positions, albeit slowly. In SPS, rigidity affects the passive and volitional range of movements just about equally. Finally, the appropriate diagnosis would have been made at the initial visit if the clinician had properly focused on the asymmetry of the patient's appendicular bradykinesia with amplitude decrement during finger tapping and reduced ipsilateral arm swing when walking. Of course, an earlier L-dopa trial would have clinched the diagnosis and prevented a misdirected work up and early treatment.

Incidentally, besides SPS, primary lateral sclerosis (PLS) and some forms of dystonia may present with severe poverty of movement (Video 3c) which may suffice to suspect them as part of the akinetic-rigid syndrome. Although these disorders are not formally listed in the differential diagnosis of parkinsonism,[9] their excessive muscle hyperactivity (which, in fact, defines SPS and dystonia as hyperkinetic disorders) leads to reduced movements (an ostensibly hypokinetic outcome) and subsequent mischaracterization as parkinsonian.

Diagnosis: Parkinson's disease (akinetic-rigid variant)

Tip: *Rigidity in PD may restrict the passive but not spontaneous range of motion. Such discrepancy is not present in SPS, with which this case was confused. Response to L-dopa is critical when doubting the parkinsonian nature of anyone with excessive rigidity.*

Case 4: Jerky hemifacial spasms

Case: This 59-year-old man presented with a 6-month history of continuous left eye blinking, upper face twitching and facial discomfort without pain. He had felt similar difficulties 3 years previously which resolved spontaneously after 3 months. The twitching was noted as having both tonic and fine myoclonic components that attenuated or disappeared during volitional tasks (Video 4a). There were no other abnormalities on the neurological or general examination. The patient was referred for consideration of botulinum toxin injections under the suspicion of hemifacial spasm (HFS).

Why should one not readily accept the diagnosis of HFS?

A subtle myoclonic component can be present at the earliest stages of HFS, usually in the periorbital region, but once spread over the ipsilateral hemi-face, the movements evolve into a mixture of tonic and myoclonic jerks rather than pure myoclonic movements. Though this patient's movements dis-appeared during speech and grinning, as demon-strated in the video, the (myo)clonic component was prominent. An epileptic disorder was sus-pected. An EEG while the patient was experiencing clinical facial twitching identified frequent epilepti-form discharges with right inferior frontal max-imum, corresponding to the facial homuncular region. Irregular epileptiform discharges or rhyth-mic/semi-rhythmic focal slowing over the right inferior frontal head region was documented during prolonged video/EEG monitoring while the patient was experiencing clinical symptoms. Carbamazepine provided almost complete resolution of the facial twitching (Video 4b). Transient recurrences of the facial twitching were documented only during periods when the patient discontinued the drug.

Discussion: Not all hemifacial spasms are HFS. What is typically considered a peripheral movement disorder can also be, as in this case, an epileptic phenomenon –epilepsia partialis continua. The epi-leptic nature of these movements was initially missed for three main reasons. First, it disappeared during sleep (though this can be the case in some forms of focal epilepsy). Second, the fine myoclonic movements were likely interpreted as post-paralytic facial myokymia, which commonly precedes or accompanies HFS.[10] And third, their disappearance with speech and other orofacial movements as may occur in some forms of dystonia,[11] assuming HFS may have been confused with focal dystonia. The

motor phenomena of focal seizures are typically not suppressed by volitional tasks.

Suspected as having isolated HFS, this patient had been referred to a movement disorders clinic for chemodenervation with botulinum toxin. How-ever, such therapeutic strategy would not have addressed the underlying pathophysiologic mech-anism, which was elucidated with EEG. With appropriate attention to phenomenologic detail, the focal spasms combining jerky and tonic fea-tures typical of HFS may be distinguishable from EPC-induced facial epileptic movements.[12]

Diagnosis: Epilepsia partialis continua mimicking hemifacial spasm.

Tip: *Atypical behaviors departing from the mixed myoclonic and tonic movements of HFS raise the possibility of an epileptic etiology. EEG should be considered in patients with isolated facial or appen-dicular movements when repetitive or intermittent myoclonus is present.*

Case 5: Paroxysmal finger posturing

Case: This 66-year-old seamstress complained of episodes of left thumb adduction and index finger extension for the last 6 months. The first such episode occurred suddenly as she was sowing a button, but subsequent episodes happened without a specific trigger. The posturing was invariably painful, lasting about 5 minutes. Their frequency had increased to about one per day. She once had cramping and stiffening of the right biceps, which "locked" her arm in an unusual position. She was referred to our attention as hand dystonia, and to consider treatment with botulinum toxin injections.

What should dampen the enthusiasm for chemodenervation?

Three main reasons: its episodic nature, their short duration, and the accompanying pain. Pain is rarely a manifestation of dystonia in any body

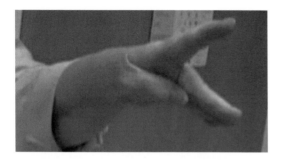

Figure 1.4. Intermittent painful hand posturing in a 66-year-old diabetic seamstress. These episodes consisted of rapid-onset painful thumb adduction, slight metacarpophalangeal flexion, and interphalangeal finger extension. These painful episodes lasted less than 5 minutes and disappeared abruptly.

distribution other than the neck. Paroxysmal posturing associated with pain can be thought of as psychogenic in nature,[13] but she had none of the episodes at the clinic, which is typically a setting when psychogenic disorders express in full bloom. In fact, she had to demonstrate what the hand posturing looked like when it occurred (Figure 1.4) (Video 5).

Is the history more exciting than the exam?

Nothing on the exam was remarkable, except for mild decreased sensation to temperature and vibration in the distal legs. She was known to have hypertension, diabetes mellitus type II, thyroid disease, chronic obstructive pulmonary disease, and obstructive sleep apnea. She was a former smoker. She was taking multiple medications for the above problems as well as vitamin D and calcium. Hence, her medical history was more intriguing than the exam and could shed light on the nature of the problem.

What does the mimicked hand posturing suggest?

Paroxysmal painful posturing of the left thumb and index finger of sudden onset and offset should remind the reader of muscle cramps rather than

dystonia, which was the initial diagnosis. The more specific combination of painful contractions of finger muscles resulting in thumb adduction, metacarpophalangeal flexion, and interphalangeal finger extension, should be recognized as tetany or carpopedal spasm (sans *pedal* [foot]; isolated carpal spasm in this case), which is a peripheral neuromuscular disorder not to be confused with dystonia.[14;15] In the absence of this particular topographical distribution, other conditions worth considering are tonic spasm of multiple sclerosis, neuromyotonia, and Lambert-Brody syndrome (exercise-induced pain, stiffness, and cramping in arm and leg muscles associated with impairment of relaxation).

In this setting, metabolic disorders of calcium, potassium, and phosphorus need to be examined. Our patient's ionized calcium was normal, but PTH and phosphorus were high and magnesium was low. Further investigations demonstrated these changes to be due to previously unrecognized renal insufficiency, likely a complication of her diabetes mellitus. Correction of the laboratory abnormalities and tighter management of her diabetes and renal insufficiency led to complete resolution of the tetany episodes.

Discussion: Tetany is classically triggered by hypocalcemia but hypomagnesemia as well as metabolic and respiratory alkalosis can also induce it.[16] Alkalotic states are capable of inducing tetany by binding calcium to proteins, thus lowering ionized calcium. In a paradoxical twist, metabolic alkalosis can also induce hypokalemia, which protects against tetany in the setting of hypocalcemia.[17] Correction of hypokalemia alone can precipitate hypocalcemic tetany.

Hypoparathyroidism is the most common cause of hypocalcemia, often as a complication of thyroid surgery or radical resection of head and neck cancers. It is confirmed when the level of parathyroid hormone (PTH) is low or inappropriately normal. Chronic hypoparathyroidism may express with *basal ganglia calcifications*.[18] This was definitely not the case here. Our patient's ionized calcium was normal, PTH was high, and she was found to have high phosphorus and low magnesium underlying early renal insufficiency, likely complications of her diabetes mellitus. When PTH is high, low serum phosphorus indicates *vitamin D deficiency or resistance* (rickets) but high phosphorus, as in this case, can be seen in *pseudohypoparathyroidism* (sporadic or autosomal dominant [Albright's osteodystrophy]), rhabdomyolysis, tumor lysis syndrome, phosphate ingestion, and renal insufficiency.[19] The latter was discovered as the reason of her decompensation. It is possible that her (pseudo) normocalcemia may have been the result of concurrent intake of vitamin D and calcium.

The peripheral nerve hyperexcitability expressed spontaneously as tetany can also be appreciated on exam through the elicitation of the classic *Chvostek's sign* (facial contraction upon tapping the skin over the facial nerve, in front of the external auditory meatus)[18] and *Trousseau's sign* (elicitation of the same carpal spasm seen in our patient when a blood pressure cuff on the patient's arm is inflated 20 mmHg above systolic blood pressure for 3–5 minutes). The management of this patient will hinge on appropriate care by a diabetes specialist and nephrologist. Certainly, antidystonic drugs or botulinum toxin should not be part of her treatment. A neurologist need be mindful that iatrogenic hypocalcemia may result from such drugs as phenobarbital, alcohol, phenytoin, carbamazepine, foscarnet, and cimetidine.

Diagnosis: Tetany or carpal spasm

Tip: *Posturing does not equal dystonia. When posturing is paroxysmal, transient, and painful, tetany should be suspected and the underlying electrolytic or acid-base disorder investigated.*

Case 6: Psychogenic tremor until proven otherwise

Contributed by Dr. Francesca Morgante, Università di Messina, Italy

Case: This 56-year-old man developed a right-hand tremor and right leg tremor rather abruptly during a financially stressful period, when he was trying to sell his house. This tremor interfered with some activities, including handwriting, to an extent that the referring physician was suspicious about a non-organic origin. Clonazepam, pramipexole, and ropinirole had been tried to no avail. There was a history of major depressive disorder with psychosis (at least 5 years prior to the onset of the movement disorder). His sister and brother suffered from a predominantly postural bilateral hand tremor of unclear nature. Examination showed a right-hand tremor at rest, on posture, and during action, which attenuated or disappeared with passive manipulation or finger tapping of the contralateral arm (Video 6a).

What features are unusual for psychogenic tremor?

Although the history, as presented, suggested a psychogenic disorder (abrupt onset, disproportionate disability to the apparent severity of the tremor) and the tremor appeared to be of similar amplitude at rest and on action, several aspects to the phenotype argued against a psychogenic etiology. First, the tremor was intermittently disrupted but never fully entrained or suppressed. Second, the intermittent right foot tremor is supported on the ground laterally rather than anteriorly, as is typical in psychogenic foot tremor (Video 6b). Third, there is a pause of the tremor on initial posture holding and a replacement of a predominantly flexion-extension tremor to a predominantly pronation-supination tremor. Finally, attention to the tremor reduces, rather than increases its amplitude.

Which alternative diagnosis and diagnostic strategy is worth pursuing?

The features listed above are highly suggestive of tremor-dominant PD. The foot involvement, particularly when unilateral, is more supportive of PD than of any other tremor disorder, excepting psychogenic, whereby a constellation of features make it highly distinctive (as shown in Video 6b). Unilateral leg tremor at onset with or without foot dystonia can be prominent at presentation for PD due to *Parkin* and *LRRK2* mutations.[20;21] In this case, genetic testing was not pursued despite this phenotypic feature and positive family history, although the results would not have been expected to influence the choice of treatment. Instead, a DaTscan was requested and found to be abnormal, supporting the clinical diagnosis of PD.

Discussion: A history of psychogenic features does not imply that the disorder is psychogenic (much as the absence of such history would not prove any disorder as organic). Despite tremor disruption or attenuation, it persisted at the same frequency and distribution throughout a variety of tasks. Although the presentation seemed abrupt, it is likely that stressful events unmasked a tremor that had been slowly developing. Unilateral tremor of psychogenic etiology may spread rapidly to a generalized or mixed distribution.[22] Spontaneous resolution and recurrence, easy distractibility together with entrainment and response to suggestion are characteristic features, which were not appreciated in this case.

Another potential pitfall relates to the reliance on ancillary testing. Although electrophysiological evaluation can be helpful where diagnostic doubt persists, it may not always fully distinguish psychogenic from organic movement disorders.[23] For example, simulated and organic propriospinal myoclonus may share a fixed pattern of muscle recruitment, synchronous activation of agonist and antagonist, electromyographic burst duration less than 1000 ms, and slow conduction in the spinal cord (5–15 m/s).[24] Although this patient had a positive DaTscan, which supported the revised clinical diagnosis, this test may yield false negatives, in which case PD may still be the underlying condition. Alternatively, a true negative DaT scan could still indicate the expected normal striatal dopamine uptake among parkinsonian patients with dopa-responsive dystonia.[25] Careful examination and appropriate interpretation of the clinical data trump potentially misleading test results.

Diagnosis: Parkinson's disease

Tip: *Historic (and sometimes electrophysiologic) features suggestive of psychogenicity do not necessarily mean the movements are psychogenic. Careful observation may reveal the presence of an organic disorder with "embellishment" or psychogenic overlay.*

REFERENCES

1. Singh S, Kumar A. Wernicke encephalopathy after obesity surgery: a systematic review. *Neurology* 2007;**68**(11):807–811.
2. Harper CG, Giles M, Finlay-Jones R. Clinical signs in the Wernicke-Korsakoff complex: a retrospective analysis of 131 cases diagnosed at necropsy. *J Neurol Neurosurg Psychiatry* 1986;**49**(4):341–345.
3. Espay AJ, Narayan RK, Duker AP, et al. Lower-body parkinsonism: reconsidering the threshold for external lumbar drainage. *Nat Clin Pract Neurol* 2008;**4**(1):50–55.
4. Matsusue E, Sugihara S, Fujii S, et al. White matter changes in elderly people: MR-pathologic correlations. Mag Reson Med Sci 2006;**5**(2):99–104.
5. Peralta C, Werner P, Holl B, et al. Parkinsonism following striatal infarcts: incidence in a prospective stroke unit cohort. *J Neural Transm* 2004;**111** (10–11):1473–1483.
6. Yamanouchi H, Nagura H. Neurological signs and frontal white matter lesions in vascular parkinsonism: a clinicopathologic study. *Stroke* 1997;**28**(5):965–969.
7. Ondo WG, Chan LL, Levy JK. Vascular parkinsonism: clinical correlates predicting motor improvement after lumbar puncture. *Mov Disord* 2002;**17**(1):91–97.
8. Steiger MJ, Thompson PD, Marsden CD. Disordered axial movement in Parkinson's disease. *J Neurol Neurosurg Psychiatry* 1996;**61**(6):645–648.
9. Poewe W, Wenning G. The differential diagnosis of Parkinson's disease. *Eur J Neurol* 2002;**9** Suppl 3:23–30.
10. Valls-Sole J, Montero J. Movement disorders in patients with peripheral facial palsy. *Mov Disord* 2003;**18**(12):1424–1435.
11. Fahn S. Clinical variants of idiopathic torsion dystonia. *J Neurol Neurosurg Psychiatry* 1989; Suppl:96–100.
12. Espay AJ, Schmithorst VJ, Szaflarski JP. Chronic isolated hemifacial spasm as a manifestation of epilepsia partialis continua. *Epilepsy Behav* 2008;**12**(2):332–336.

13. Lang AE. Psychogenic dystonia: a review of 18 cases. *Can J Neurol Sci* 1995;**22**(2):136–143.

14. Athappan G, Ariyamuthu VK. Images in clinical medicine: Chvostek's sign and carpopedal spasm. *N Engl J Med* 2009;**360**(18):e24.

15. Matustik MC. Late-onset tetany with hypocalcemia and hyperphosphatemia. *Am J Dis Child* 1986;**140**(9): 854–855.

16. Weiss-Guillet EM, Takala J, Jakob SM. Diagnosis and management of electrolyte emergencies. *Best Pract Res Clin Endocrinol Metab* 2003;**17**(4):623–651.

17. Dickerson RN. Treatment of hypocalcemia in critical illness – part 1. *Nutrition* 2007;**23**(4):358–361.

18. Narayan SK, Sivaprasad P, Sahoo RN, et al. Teaching video NeuroImage: Chvostek sign with Fahr syndrome in a patient with hypoparathyroidism. *Neurology* 2008;**71**(24):e79.

19. Moe SM. Disorders involving calcium, phosphorus, and magnesium. *Prim Care* 2008;**35**(2):215–2vi.

20. Klein C, Pramstaller PP, Kis B, et al. Parkin deletions in a family with adult-onset, tremor-dominant parkinsonism: expanding the phenotype. *Ann Neurol* 2000;**48**(1):65–71.

21. Khan NL, Jain S, Lynch JM, et al. Mutations in the gene LRRK2 encoding dardarin (PARK8) cause familial Parkinson's disease: clinical, pathological, olfactory and functional imaging and genetic data. *Brain* 2005;**128**(Pt 12):2786–2796.

22. Kim YJ, Pakiam AS, Lang AE. Historical and clinical features of psychogenic tremor: a review of 70 cases. *Can J Neurol Sci* 1999;**26**(3):190–195.

23. Gupta A, Lang AE. Psychogenic movement disorders. 2009;**22**(4):430–436.

24. Kang SY, Sohn YH. Electromyography patterns of pro-priospinal myoclonus can be mimicked voluntarily. *Mov Disord* 2006;**21**(8):1241–1244.

25. Marshall V, Grosset D. Role of dopamine transporter imaging in routine clinical practice. *Mov Disord* 2003;**18**(12):1415–1423.

2

Attributing findings to a known or suspected disorder

Case 7: Mild spasticity in the stiff-person syndrome

Case: A 57-year-old man began to have episodes of left leg stiffness and falls about 6 years prior to presentation at our office. His leg stiffness progressed to the point of limiting his tennis playing and ultimately requiring temporary use of a cane. As part of his evaluation for these symptoms, anti-glutamic acid decarboxylase (anti-GAD-65) antibody level was reportedly extremely high, above 45 000 U/mL. A diagnosis of stiff-person syndrome (SPS) was made. He markedly improved within 2 weeks of initiating treatment with diazepam. This level of response was maintained although requiring progressively higher doses (5 mg every morning and 10 mg at bedtime). He did well for most of the subsequent 4 to 5 years. Then, he started to note intermittent episodes of additional stiffness in the left leg and had a fall. He also complained of mild numbness in the right leg, which was the only symptom he endorsed outside his left leg. His gait, however, looked relatively normal, and during his first examination in the office he had to imitate how bad it could truly get (Video 7a).

Can we attribute the reported worsening of his gait to his known SPS?

Although confirming SPS by repeating anti-GAD antibody testing was warranted, the examination had unusual features for this disorder. The patient showed generalized hyperreflexia, sans jaw jerk, with spasticity, ankle clonus, and left Babinski (Video 7b). Although hyperreflexia is an acceptable upper motor neuron sign in SPS, its presence everywhere (even if sparing the jaw) is not. Furthermore, any upper motor sign other than hyperreflexia is exclusionary for the diagnosis of SPS.[1]

What do the neurological findings suggest? What should we do next?

Despite a confirmed increase of anti-GAD-65 antibodies on repeat testing (16 768.0 U/mL [Normal, 0.0–1.5]) and prior record of excellent response to diazepam, the new set of findings extended beyond the accepted phenotypic spectrum of SPS and suggested the presence of a concurrent cervical myelopathy, possibly due to spinal stenosis or complicated disc herniation. Indeed, a cervical spine MRI showed a bilobed C6-C7 disc herniation causing flattening and abnormal signal within the left anterior spinal cord.

What should be done next?

Two spinal cord disorders are present: an autoimmune encephalomyelopathy (SPS) and a cervical compressive myelopathy. A cautious approach would be to "treat" the high anti-GAD levels by increasing the dose of diazepam to a new target of 20 mg/day, even though the levels of anti-GAD antibodies are unreliable predictors of response to therapy.[2] If this approach fails to prevent progression, surgical resolution of the cervical disc herniation becomes desirable.

Discussion: SPS refers to the combination of rigidity, reflex and action-induced spasms, and continuous motor unit activity at rest due to impairment in the production of GABA. Rigidity is the key finding. Rigidity is also a key finding in disorders of glycine. Glycine can be impaired presynaptically (tetanus), post-synaptically (strychnine), or due to mutations in the glycine receptor (hyperekplexia). In these disorders, rigidity is pure, that is, there is no intrusion of the velocity-dependent hypertonia we refer to as spasticity.[3] Spasms are rapid in hyperekplexia or tetanus, corresponding to glycine-mediated fast inhibitory post-synaptic potentials, and less abrupt in SPS patients, consistent with GABA-mediated slow inhibitory post-synaptic potentials. The rigidity in this patient may be within the spectrum of SPS but the upper motor neuron findings beyond hyperreflexia suggested corticospinal involvement.[4] Besides these findings, other exclusionary features for the diagnosis of SPS include lower motor neuron signs, sphincter and sensory disturbances, and cognitive impairment. Unlike the more common forms of SPS, patients like ours with the stiff-limb syndrome variant have less evidence of autoimmune diseases, no involvement of truncal musculature, and tend to have a better prognosis.[5]

A final word related to the value of anti-GAD antibody titers and associated disorders. Markedly high titers, such as those documented in this patient, are only recognized in two disorders: SPS and cerebellar ataxia. Low titers, in contrast, are seen in adult-onset drug-refractory epilepsy, type I diabetes mellitus, and other autoimmune endocrinopathies such as Graves' disease and pernicious anemia. Taken together, up to 80% of SPS patients have a personal or family history of autoimmune disorders, either endocrine or rheumatologic (systemic lupus erythematosus, rheumatoid arthritis, and vitiligo).[6]

Diagnosis: Stiff-person syndrome and concurrent cervical myelopathy

Tip: *Hyperreflexia is the only upper motor neuron sign allowable in SPS. Spasticity should suggest concurrent corticospinal tract involvement, such as that derived from compressive cervical myelopathy.*

Case 8: Unsteadiness when standing

Case: An 82-year-old woman noted "weakness" and numbness in both legs, as well as lightheadedness when standing over several years. The latency between standing and unsteadiness had shortened progressively. Walking decreased the unsteadiness and sitting completely resolved it. Recently discovered orthostatic hypotension had been corrected by an admission for intravenous hydration, without improvement in her symptoms. Examination showed previously unrecognized mild dementia (MMSE = 25/30, Frontal Assessment Battery = 15/18; Montreal Cognitive Assessment = 19/30) and unsteadiness when standing (Video 8a). The initial assessment note documented mild isolated iliopsoas weakness, which was attributed to deconditioning and a "palpable leg tremor that worsened with stationary standing and attenuated with walking and sitting, and can be transferred to the arms when supporting weight on them."

Where is this examiner leading the reader? What is the pitfall?

The story is highly suggestive of orthostatic tremor, a unique high-frequency (14– to 16 Hz) tremor of weight-bearing limbs. The examiner's note is leading to this foregone conclusion. However, palpation or auscultation of a high-frequency repetitive or oscillatory activity in the limbs is a notoriously unreliable method to discriminate any frequency greater than 8 Hz. Despite a compelling story for orthostatic tremor, one must acknowledge the limitations of neurological examination and admit that an alternative orthostatic disorder is also possible. The major pitfall here is in assuming the story was clear enough to merit circumventing a necessary diagnostic step in this type of manifestation: electrophysiology.

How does electrophysiology help?

In fact, surface EMG recorded from both tibialis anterior and gastrocnemius muscles failed to confirm the suspected tremor (Figure 2.1). Instead of

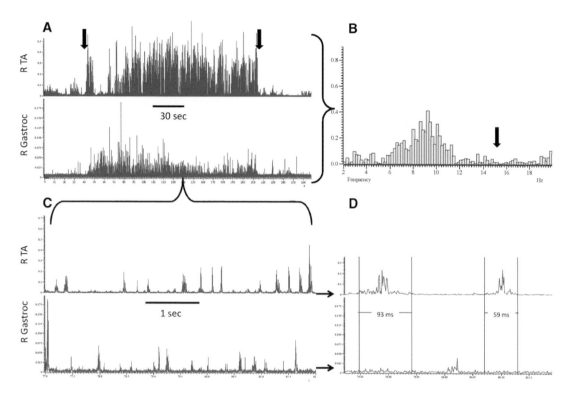

Figure 2.1. Raw surface EMG (A) of the right tibialis anterior (R TA) and gastrocnemius (R Gastroc) shows normal increase in amplitude when standing (between vertical arrows). Power spectrum analysis between these muscles (B) showed no coherence at the 14–16 Hz range (single vertical arrow), as expected in orthostatic tremor. Inspection of the raw EMG (C) indeed revealed non-rhythmic activity, with individual bursts (D) lasting < 150 ms, within the range for myoclonus.

repetitive, oscillatory activity, there were random, non-rhythmic bursts of EMG activity, ranging from 50 to 130 ms in duration. This activity was present in the sampled leg muscles when standing, and disappeared when sitting. Coherence analysis showed lack of synchrony between the right and left legs. These findings ruled out orthostatic tremor and confirmed a phenotypically similar but pathophysiologically distinct entity: orthostatic myoclonus.

Discussion: This patient had been appropriately thought of as having orthostatic hypotension first (which may have been present early on) and orthostatic tremor later. However, without electrophysiology the correct diagnosis of orthostatic

myoclonus would have been missed. Compared to orthostatic myoclonus, the positional orthostatic tremor tends to have a topographical involvement beyond the legs (Video 8b) and may bear greater relationship to mechanisms that modulate weight bearing or the perception of upward force applied to the legs.[7;8] It has been suggested that patients with orthostatic myoclonus could be considered as having "apraxia" or "gait initiation difficulty," with leg jerking that may not be clinically apparent, only revealed with electrophysiology.[9] Orthostatic myoclonus may develop in the background of neurodegenerative diseases, such as Parkinson's disease, MSA, DLB, Alzheimer's disease, and cerebral amyloid angiopathy.[9;10] The most common diagnoses with which orthostatic myoclonus may be

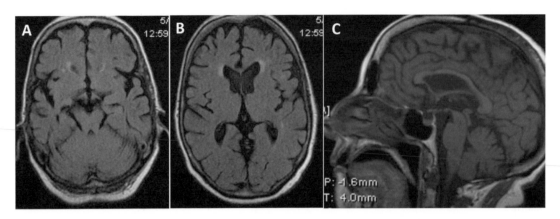

Figure 2.2. Axial FLAIR brain MRI sequences at the midbrain (A) and thalamic (B) levels showing mild temporal- and frontal-predominant cortical atrophy; mid-sagittal T1-weighted MRI (C) demonstrates mild thinning of the body and genu of the corpus callosum with relative preservation of the splenium, suggesting a reduction of interhemispheric frontotemporal fibers.

confused are normal pressure hydrocephalus and, fittingly, orthostatic tremor.[9] Clonazepam can be helpful to both orthostatic disorders, though its efficacy is typically suboptimal.

Diagnosis: Orthostatic myoclonus

Tip: *Surface electromyography is indispensable to distinguish the orthostatic disorders, orthostatic tremor and myoclonus.*

Case 9: Supranuclear gaze palsy and parkinsonism: why not PSP?

Case: A 70-year-old woman suffered backward falls and shortly thereafter slowed and hypophonic voice, word-finding difficulty, trouble reading, dysphagia, and generalized weakness. Examination at 9 months after symptom onset demonstrated dementia (MMSE = 15/30; Frontal Assessment Battery = 8/18; abnormal clock drawing test), non-fluent aphasia with agrammatism and impaired repetition, pseudo-bulbar affect, supranuclear vertical gaze paresis, apraxia of eyelid closing, frontal release signs, diffuse hyperreflexia and limb weakness, and marked postural and gait impairment (Video 9). Brain MRI showed mild cortical atrophy, predominantly

affecting frontal and temporal lobes (Figure 2.2). EMG of the lower extremities revealed widespread fibrillations. She died of bronchopneumonia 14 months after symptom onset.

If this is a progressive supranuclear palsy phenotype why isn't it PSP?

Although the phenotype (early falls, parkinsonism, supranuclear gaze paresis) is clearly suggestive of PSP, neither the time course nor the "extra" features would support the PSP diagnosis. A disease course of 14 months qualifies it as rapidly progressive. In this context, moderate dementia with severe language deficits arising early on and weakness with early pyramidal signs are exclusionary for the clinical diagnosis of possible or probable PSP.[11]

What PSP-like disorders do we have to think about?

Atypical PSP or PSP-like presentations include pure akinesia syndrome, primary progressive freezing of gait, corticobasal syndrome, and frontotemporal dementia. The non-degenerative category includes multi-infarct state, mesencephalic tumors, Whipple's disease, Niemann-Pick disease type C, neurosyphilis, and mitochondrial myopathy. In this case, three clinical clues should have helped steer the diagnosis to the appropriate syndrome: the language impairment categorized as progressive non-fluent aphasia (PNFA) and the fronto-temporal pattern of atrophy on brain MRI suggest the language presentation of frontotemporal dementia (FTD), the clinical syndrome, or frontotemporal lobar degeneration (FTLD), the neuropathologic correlate. The addition of weakness with hyperreflexia on exam and fibrillations on EMG also suggests the presence of motor neuron disease (MND). Hence, this combination would be best reported as FTLD-MND with a PSP-like presentation. The MND component explains the rapid decline.

Discussion: This case was pathologically confirmed as FTLD-MND due to TDP-43 proteinopathy (without progranulin mutation).[12] This tremorless, hypokinetic-rigid syndrome with early falls and oculomotor impairment developing in the context of severe language deficits has also been labeled PSP-PNFA. Severe language deficits are considered exclusionary for the diagnosis of PSP and should force the consideration of PSP-like disorders falling in the frontotemporal dementia–parkinsonism spectrum.[13] A PSP-like presentation with MND can occur in the setting of an underlying tauopathy ("atypical PSP with corticospinal degeneration")[14] or TDP-43 proteinopathy.[15] Parkinsonian phenotypes with frontal-predominant dementia have been considered highly predictive of tau-positive neuropathology.[16;17] The tauopathies (FTLD-tau) are associated with the accumulation of hyperphosphorylated tau and include Pick's disease, PSP, CBD, argyrophilic grain disease, multiple system tauopathy with presenile dementia, and white matter tauopathy with globular glial inclusions.[18]

Besides FTLD-MND, rapidly progressive dementia with parkinsonism has been reported in cases of Alzheimer's disease, DLB, CBD, PSP, and CJD.[19] FTLD is the most common anatomic correlate of progressive frontotemporal dementia and parkinsonism, more so if language is involved. The addition of MND ultimately helped narrow the differential diagnosis significantly in this case. Unfortunately, no available treatment could alleviate any of this patient's symptoms.

Diagnosis: FTLD-MND with a PSP-like presentation

Tip: *PSP and corticobasal syndrome are recognized phenotypes of FTLD. Suspect FTLD when these presentations are "contaminated" with early dysexecutive dementia, language impairment, and/or personality disorders.*

Case 10: Chronic hemifacial pain and tightness

Case: This 40-year-old woman dated the onset of her problems to the time immediately after the delivery of her first child, 4 years ago, when she developed post-partum eclampsia as well as migraines, partly experienced as "rubber bands being flicked." The migraines were sharp, located in the right retroorbital region, and radiated to the temporal and ipsilateral jaw region. During these events, she felt painful tightness of the right facial muscles (Video 10a). Evaluation at the time led to the diagnosis of temporomandibular joint pain, and an orthotic device was placed in her jaw. This procedure was followed by symptomatic improvement but she ultimately experienced recurrence and worsening of the muscle pain. Botulinum toxin injections into the masseters, temporalis, splenius capitis, and trapezius were initially successful at relieving the pain but their efficacy decreased over time. Excessive contractions of jaw muscles were felt to represent adult-onset oromandibular dystonia and re-exposure to a higher total dose of botulinum toxin to selected right-sided muscles (including but perhaps not limited to the temporalis, masseters, and trapezius) was suggested.

What elements of the history do not fit with the suspected disorder?

First, pain in craniofacial dystonia is very rare (cervical dystonia is the exception to the no-pain rule of dystonias). Second, the symptoms are equally intense at rest and during action (dystonia is mostly induced or exacerbated by action and, with few exceptions, relieved or attenuated with rest). Third, the association with migraine is unusual and a tight correlation between these processes is rarely seen in dystonia. Nevertheless, a larger dose of botulinum toxin type A (Botox, 60 units) was injected into the right masseter and temporalis with additional injections (40 units) given to the right splenius capitis and trapezius. The affected area continued to experience as much pain and tightness.

What may still be missing to clarify the diagnosis and redress her management?

An EMG of the most affected muscles, the right masseter and temporalis. The study revealed spontaneous recurring mono- and polysynaptic discharges. The monosynaptic discharges occurred at 20–30 Hz (Video 10b). The left masseter muscle was normal. Together with the symptoms, these continuous simple and complex discharges recorded from muscles innervated by the right trigeminal nerve were diagnostic of hemimasticatory spasm (HMS). Other treatment options were discussed, including alternative chemodenervation toxins, clonazepam, and carbamazepine. Treatment with carbamazepine markedly alleviated her symptoms.

Discussion: HMS is a rare facial movement disorder characterized by isolated and sustained muscle contraction of masticatory muscles due to hyperexcitability of the motor branch of the trigeminal nerve. Though most cases are idiopathic, HMS may occur as a complication of pontine infarctions affecting the trigeminal nucleus[20] or in association with progressive facial hemiatrophy and localized scleroderma.[21] Lacking these historical and clinical clues, this patient's symptoms were incorrectly considered to represent oromandibular dystonia. However, a constantly painful and much localized process, not causing overt movements, was unlikely to have been dystonia. The EMG established the diagnosis by demonstrating ectopic excitation of the trigeminal motor root (or its nucleus), an abnormality analogous to the ectopic excitation of

the facial nerve in hemifacial spasm.[22;23] The relatively rapid appearance of HMS around pregnancy has been previously reported and may be a clinical pearl for this diagnosis.[24] Reported treatment options in HFS include botulinum toxin injections, clonazepam, carbamazepine and, in refractory cases, selective surgical denervation of trigeminal nerve branches.

Diagnosis: Hemimasticatory spasm

Tip: *Hemimasticatory spasm has a distinct history, phenomenology, and EMG pattern but can be misdiagnosed as oromandibular dystonia or temporomandibular joint pain. HMS is, electrophysiologically, similar to hemifacial spasm but restricted to the masseter and temporalis muscles.*

Case 11: Anxiety in Parkinson's disease: dopaminergic wearing off?

Case: This 74-year-old woman with Parkinson's disease for 8 years, starting with left arm resting tremor, followed by hypophonia, micrographia, anosmia, and urinary frequency, went on to develop motor complications with wearing off and peak-dose, L-dopa-induced upper-body dyskinesias. Her exquisite sensitivity to L-dopa required small 25 mg titration increments during the efforts to mitigate the motor fluctuations. She started to develop increasing episodes of anxiety, associated with excesssive fatigue and palpitations, especially after meals. These were interpreted as representing end-of-dose non-motor fluctuations and were addressed, sequentially, by decreasing the interdose interval and increasing the individual doses of L-dopa. Anxiety would seem to abate somewhat with this strategy, although at the expense of worsening dyskinesias. The episodes of anxiety continued to be present despite efforts at minimizing the off periods with COMT- and MAO-B-inhibitors. Lorazepam was introduced to ameliorate these symptoms and minimize the need for fruitless evaluations in the emergency department.

Why is this problem not resolving with efforts at decreasing the wearing-off periods?

Three potential reasons: anxiety may be primarily non-dopaminergic in nature, it may respond to a separate process and bear no relationship to L-dopa pharmacokinetics, or it may be an idiosyncratic consequence of exposure to one of her medications. When she was dyskinetic, fewer episodes of anxiety were perceived. As such, the palpitations were interpreted as representing wearing-off non-motor fluctuations in the form of panic attacks. Higher doses of L-dopa were, however, not tolerated because she felt "more nervous" and certainly more dyskinetic.

Could a specialized consultation help resolve this problem?

Not by examining the psychiatric underpinnings of her anxiety but the palpitations that were believed to be its byproduct. Indeed, a cardiologist obtained a 24-hour Holter, which demonstrated paroxysmal atrial fibrillations. With the supervision of her cardiologist, the antiarrhythmic flecainide was introduced and the dose of L-dopa was judiciously lowered, with optimal control of both the anxiety episodes and her motor function.

Discussion: Arrhythmias are one of the least appreciated complications of L-dopa therapy,[25] less common but just as disabling as hallucinations, orthostatic hypotension, depression, or even dyskinesias.[26] "Palpitations or arrhythmias" were listed as occurring in 7.5% of the PD cohort reported by Barbeau on his seminal experience during the first decade of L-dopa treatment (as a comparison, dyskinesias are reported in 50%, nausea or vomiting in 44%, hypotension in 31%, and hallucinations or vivid dreams in 16%).[27] Admittedly, in Barbeau's time L-dopa was given without a dopa decarboxylase inhibitor. The addition of carbidopa (or benserazide in Europe) to the L-dopa formulation should have made the risk of arrhythmias much less common, even if vigilance in the setting of refractory "anxiety" remains necessary. This is fortunate

since discontinuing L-dopa is not an option for most patients experiencing side effects. The uncovering of L-dopa-induced arrhythmias such as paroxysmal atrial fibrillations or premature ventricular contractions warrants the introduction of an antiarrhythmic to the treatment regimen.[28] Anxiety can also be the result of peak-dose and wearing-off phenomena to L-dopa. This mechanism may have also been present early on, falsely reassuring the treating clinician that an early and partial anti-anxiety effect from the higher-L-dopa treatment approach had been effective.

Diagnosis: L-dopa-induced arrhythmia in a PD patient

Tip: *Although a common non-motor fluctuation, "anxiety" can also be uncommonly due to L-dopa induced arrhythmias. Its persistence despite efforts at mitigating the off-on fluctuations warrants a cardiology consultation.*

Case 12: Ataxia and a "gray zone" genetic test

Case: This 63-year-old man was evaluated for progressive unsteadiness. Three years previously he had an episode of vertigo associated with nausea and vomiting, which resolved spontaneously. A year later, he began to develop slowly progressive unsteadiness when walking and clumsiness with fine motor tasks. Within the last year, he started falling eventually up to once per month, mostly sideways, especially as his steps were "not landing evenly on the ground." He had been relying on a cane for the last month. His speech had become slurred and he was choking on liquids, especially hot ones. He had some urinary urgency and rare episodes of urinary incontinence.

He had been recently diagnosed with hepatitis C and reported that treatment with interferon made his balance much better but this intervention was stopped due to the induction of low white blood cell count. Also, as a former worker in a printing company, he reported exposure to

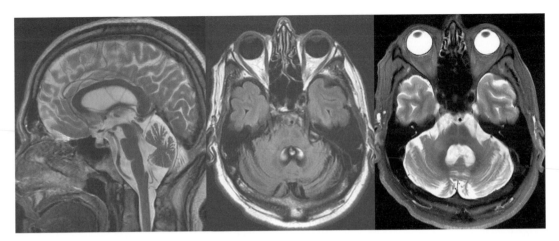

Figure 2.3. Mid-sagittal T2-weighted and axial T2-weighted and FLAIR brain MRI sequences at the level of the pons showing an olivopontocerebellar pattern of atrophy with prominent "hot-cross bun" sign. Squint some and a high signal emerges in the right middle cerebellar peduncle.

hydrochloric acid, muriatic acid, nitric acid, copper sulfate, and chromic acid for over two decades. Finally, his family history was remarkable in that a brother, a maternal female cousin, and one of her sister's daughters had childhood-onset mental retardation.

Which of the above clues should the clinician hold on to? Which to disregard?

Progressive unsteadiness, dysphagia, and mild neurogenic bladder in the background of hepatitis C, potentially toxic exposures, and an intriguing family history bode poorly for an attention-challenged, time-constrained clinician. The two conditions that rapidly spring to mind *beg* for some tremor in the picture: acquired hepatolenticular degeneration (assuming hepatitis C has caused liver cirrhosis) and fragile X tremor-ataxia syndrome (assuming the lack of a clear X-linked pattern of inheritance of mental retardation is a disposable matter). Finally, there is no knowledge on the intensity and neurotropism of the toxic exposures volunteered by this patient, but there is always room for endorsing a novel neurotoxic syndrome.

Does the examination help?

He showed a predominantly truncal ataxia and hypermetric saccades but no peripheral neuropathy, pyramidal dysfunction, or overt cognitive impairment (Montreal Cognitive Assessment = 26/30), suggesting a pure cerebellar ataxia, perhaps with a touch of parkinsonism (Video 12). There was definitely no tremor in the phenotype.

Do the brain MRI and a few "hot" genetic tests help?

The brain MRI showed marked atrophy of the medulla, pons, and cerebellum, a pattern often described as olivo-ponto-cerebellar atrophy (OPCA). A "hot-cross bun" sign is readily appreciated (Figure 2.3). Sporadic OPCA most often implies MSA-C.[29;30] But if this family history can be made to fit –and your eye-squinting exercise confirms the "MCP sign"– perhaps one could sell this case as a tremorless form of fragile X tremor-ataxia syndrome (FTAS). Finally, a paraneoplastic disorder could be considered, although a 3-year course seems too long.

The *FMR1* (fragile site mental retardation 1 gene) mutation testing revealed 47 CGG repeats in the

FMR1 gene, within the "gray zone" (40–54 repeats) for FXTAS (55–200 repeats).

Discussion: There was a strong temptation to ascribe this patient's picture of progressive cerebellar ataxia and dysautonomia to a "gray zone" FXTAS when in fact it is perfectly consistent with MSA-C. From a clinical perspective, both tremor and cognitive impairment, fundamental components of FXTAS, are absent here. From an imaging perspective, the "hot-cross bun sign" has never been reported in FXTAS nor has the subtle high signal at the MCP of the magnitude reported in this condition. Furthermore, FXTAS induces generalized brain atrophy rather than atrophy restricted to the brainstem and cerebellum, as well as more white matter changes.[31] Importantly, the family history of mental retardation is not consistent with the expected X-linked pattern of inheritance for fragile X syndrome, whereby only boys should be affected. Finally, the rate of FMRI premutation among MSA-C cases is very low, between 0.1 and 0.5%, slightly above the population rate and there are no data on "gray zone" repeats.[32] Importantly, no *FMR1* premutation carriers were identified among 81 screened patients with pathologically proven MSA.[33] Hence, the perfectly round hole of MSA-C in this case does not accept the square peg of gray zone FXTAS.

Diagnosis: Cerebellar variant of multiple system atrophy (MSA-C)

Tip: *Genetic testing for FXTAS should not be performed routinely in cases fulfilling criteria for MSA. A "gray zone" genetic test report can lead the clinician to the wrong conclusion. Sporadic OPCA with a hot-cross bun sign, in the setting of cerebellar ataxia and dysautonomia, should suggest MSA-C.*

REFERENCES

1. Espay AJ, Chen R. Rigidity and spasms from autoimmune encephalomyelopathies: stiff-person syndrome. *Muscle Nerve* 2006;**34**(6):677–690.

2. Meinck HM, Thompson PD. Stiff man syndrome and related conditions. *Mov Disord* 2002;**17**(5):853–866.

3. Siegler EL, Beck LH. Stiffness: a pathophysiologic approach to diagnosis and treatment. *J Gen Intern Med* 1989;**4**(6):533–540.

4. Wilson RK, Murinson BB. Sudden spasms following gradual lordosis – the stiff-person syndrome. *Nat Clin Pract Neurol* 2006;**2**(8):455–459.

5. Barker RA, Revesz T, Thom M, et al. Review of 23 patients affected by the stiff man syndrome: clinical subdivision into stiff trunk (man) syndrome, stiff limb syndrome, and progressive encephalomyelitis with rigidity. *J Neurol Neurosurg Psychiatry* 1998;**65**(5):633–640.

6. Dalakas MC, Fujii M, Li M, et al. The clinical spectrum of anti-GAD antibody-positive patients with stiff-person syndrome. *Neurology* 2000;**55**(10):1531–1535.

7. Piboolnurak P, Yu QP, Pullman SL. Clinical and neurophysiologic spectrum of orthostatic tremor: case series of 26 subjects. *Mov Disord* 2005;**20**(11):1455–1461.

8. Gerschlager W, Brown P. Myoclonus. *Curr Opin Neurol* 2009;**22**(4):414–418.

9. Glass GA, Ahlskog JE, Matsumoto JY. Orthostatic myoclonus: a contributor to gait decline in selected elderly. *Neurology* 2007;**68**(21):1826–1830.

10. Leu-Semenescu S, Roze E, Vidailhet M, et al. Myoclonus or tremor in orthostatism: an under-recognized cause of unsteadiness in Parkinson's disease. *Mov Disord* 2007;**22**(14):2063–2069.

11. Litvan I, Agid Y, Calne D, et al. Clinical research criteria for the diagnosis of progressive supranuclear palsy (Steele-Richardson-Olszewski syndrome): report of the NINDS-SPSP international workshop. *Neurology* 1996;**47**(1):1–9.

12. Espay AJ, Spina S, Houghton DJ, et al. Rapidly progressive atypical parkinsonism associated with frontotemporal lobar degeneration and motor neuron disease. *J Neurol Neurosurg Psychiatry* 2011;**82**:751–753.

13. Espay AJ, Litvan I. Parkinsonism and frontotemporal dementia: the clinical overlap. *J Mol Neurosci* 2011;**45**(3):343–349.

14. Josephs KA, Katsuse O, Beccano-Kelly DA, et al. Atypical progressive supranuclear palsy with corticospinal tract degeneration. *J Neuropathol Exp Neurol* 2006;**65**(4):396–405.

15. Paviour DC, Lees AJ, Josephs KA, et al. Frontotemporal lobar degeneration with ubiquitin-only-immunoreactive neuronal changes: broadening the clinical picture to

include progressive supranuclear palsy. *Brain* 2004;**127** (Pt 11):2441–2451.

16. Hodges JR, Davies RR, Xuereb JH, et al. Clinicopathological correlates in frontotemporal dementia. *Ann Neurol* 2004;**56**(3):399–406.

17. Josephs KA, Petersen RC, Knopman DS, et al. Clinicopathologic analysis of frontotemporal and corticobasal degenerations and PSP. *Neurology* 2006;**66**(1):41–48.

18. Cairns NJ, Bigio EH, Mackenzie IR, et al. Neuropathologic diagnostic and nosologic criteria for frontotemporal lobar degeneration: consensus of the Consortium for Frontotemporal Lobar Degeneration. *Acta Neuropathol (Berl)* 2007;**114**(1):5–22.

19. Josephs KA, Ahlskog JE, Parisi JE, et al. Rapidly progressive neurodegenerative dementias. *Arch Neurol* 2009;**66**(2):201–207.

20. Gunduz A, Karaali-Savrun F, Uluduz D. Hemimasticatory spasm following pontine infarction. *Mov Disord* 2007;**22**(11):1674–1675.

21. Kim HJ, Jeon BS, Lee KW. Hemimasticatory spasm associated with localized scleroderma and facial hemiatrophy. *Arch Neurol* 2000;**57**(4):576–580.

22. Auger RG, Litchy WJ, Cascino TL, et al. Hemimasticatory spasm: clinical and electrophysiologic observations. *Neurology* 1992;**42**(12):2263–2266.

23. Thompson PD, Carroll WM. Hemimasticatory and hemifacial spasm: a common pathophysiology? *Clin Exp Neurol* 1983;**19**:110–119.

24. Cersosimo MG, Bertoti A, Roca CU, et al. Botulinum toxin in a case of hemimasticatory spasm with severe worsening during pregnancy. *Clin Neuropharmacol* 2004;**27**(1):6–8.

25. Goldberg LI, Whitsett TL. Cardiovascular effects of levodopa. *Clin Pharmacol Ther* 1971;**12**(2):376–382.

26. Jenkins RB, Mendelson SH, Lamid S, et al. Levodopa therapy of patients with Parkinsonism and heart disease. *Br Med J* 1972;**3**(5825):512–514.

27. Barbeau A. L-dopa therapy in Parkinson's disease: a critical review of nine years' experience. *Can Med Assoc J* 1969;**101**(13):59–68.

28. Mars H, Krall J. L-dopa and cardiac arrhythmias. *N Engl J Med* 1971;**285**(25):1437.

29. Schrag A, Good CD, Miszkiel K, et al. Differentiation of atypical parkinsonian syndromes with routine MRI. *Neurology* 2000;**54**(3):697–702.

30. Massano J, Costa F, Nadais G. Teaching neuroImage: MRI in multiple system atrophy: "hot cross bun" sign and hyperintense rim bordering the putamina. *Neurology* 2008;**71**(15):e38.

31. Leehey MA. Fragile X-associated tremor/ataxia syndrome: clinical phenotype, diagnosis, and treatment. *J Investig Med* 2009;**57**(8):830–836.

32. Biancalana V, Toft M, Le Ber I, et al. FMR1 premutations associated with fragile X-associated tremor/ataxia syndrome in multiple system atrophy. *Arch Neurol* 2005;**62**(6):962–966.

33. Kamm C, Healy DG, Quinn NP, et al. The fragile X tremor-ataxia syndrome in the differential diagnosis of multiple system atrophy: data from the EMSA Study Group. *Brain* 2005;**128**(Pt 8):1855–1860.

3

Clinical findings that are subtle

Case 13: Orofacial dystonia in presumed PD

Case: Four years ago, this 65-year-old man began having trouble with his left foot while trying to keep up with the clog dancing lessons he was teaching. Within the next 2 years, in addition to worsening of his left foot clumsiness, he developed poor balance when dancing as well as left hand tremor when bringing the left arm to his ears. He had a fall 3 years into his symptoms, precipitated by his left foot getting "stuck to the ground." At that point, left hand rest tremor and hypophonia were fully declared, cognitive function was normal, and the diagnosis of Parkinson's disease was made (Video 13a).

Were there historic features that would have raised some concern as to this diagnosis?

A fall within 3 years is somewhat concerning. Tremor and walking improved with L-dopa, but benefits quickly eroded. Subsequent dose increases generated nausea, fatigue, and worsened his postural lightheadedness. He had had erectile dysfunction, orthostatic hypotension, and dream enactment behaviors during his sleep for several years. Although all of these comorbidities can predate and accompany PD, it was the orofacial movements that were documented at a follow-up visit, which decidedly steered the diagnostic impression away from PD (Video 13b). Although he was mostly unaware of these, and there was no clear relationship of this behavior to the dose cycle,

he acknowledged that his jaw felt tighter when the dose of L-dopa would otherwise "kick in."

Does this development alone change the diagnostic impression?

Although L-dopa-induced orofacial dystonia can be seen in PD, it is a recognized red flag in parkinsonism, pointing in the direction of multiple system atrophy. Indeed, by the sixth year of symptoms, he had developed moderate to severe balance problems and falls, several backward. His orthostatic hypotension had become a challenge, despite increased fluids and salt as well as a combination of midodrine and fludrocortisone. In addition to his erectile dysfunction, he had more episodes of urinary urgency, frequency, and incontinence. The worsening in postural reflexes and dysautonomia, and insufficient response to L-dopa had made it clear that the diagnosis needed revision in favor of MSA. A brain MRI was highly supportive of this diagnosis (Figure 3.1).

Discussion: MSA is probably more commonly misdiagnosed as PD than any other atypical parkinsonism. This is likely due to an early clinical picture that often includes a "reassuring" asymmetric resting tremor and no cognitive impairment but also because the early presence of dysautonomia can be congruent with the broad phenotypic spectrum of PD. Beyond a fall earlier than is typical for PD (within 3 years), the subtle but unusual topographic distribution of his L-dopa-induced orofacial dyskinesias, which was largely dystonic, was the more

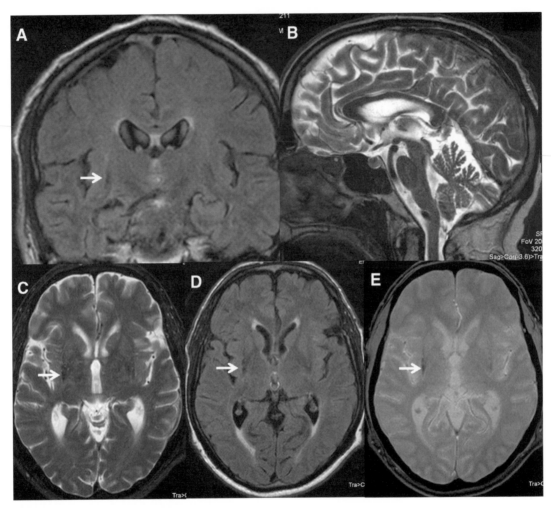

Figure 3.1. Coronal FLAIR (A), mid-sagittal T2-weighted (B), and axial T2-weighted (C), FLAIR (D), and T2* gradient echo (E) brain MRI sequences showing atrophy of the right posterolateral putamen (contralateral to the more affected side) and cerebellar vermis. These findings are highly supportive of the clinical diagnosis of the parkinsonian variant of multiple system atrophy (MSA-P).

telling development in favor of a diagnosis of MSA. In full bloom, this manifestation has earned the descriptor of "risus sardonicus" (sardonic grin) given the marked involvement of orofacial and platysma musculature, reminiscent of cephalic tetanus.[1] Its induction or worsening by action (speech, particularly) and its abatement with sensory tricks suggest the orofacial dyskinesia of MSA is a

predominantly dystonic complication of L-dopa (Video 13c), although it has also been documented in L-dopa naïve patients.[2] Wenning and colleagues have proposed that the generation of this orofacial complication results from selective sparing of ventral striatopallidal circuitry,[1] also supported by evidence that stimulation of ventral striatal dopamine release induces orofacial choreodystonia in rats.[3]

Table 3.1. Historical and examination features that best distinguish MSA from PD

Historical features	Examination features
Early instability with recurrent falls (within 3 years of disease onset)*	Orofacial dystonia
Rapid progression ("wheelchair sign": dependent < 10 years from disease onset)	Early camptocormia (prolonged episodes of forward trunk flexion); later appearance is more common in PD
"Contractures" (or dystonia) of hands or feet**	Pisa syndrome (prolonged episodes of lateral trunk flexion)
REM sleep behavior disorder (dream enactment behaviors)	Disproportionate antecollis (severe neck flexion, minor flexion elsewhere)
Sleep apnea, excessive snoring	Myoclonic tremor (irregular postural or action tremor of the hands and/or fingers)
Cold hands/feet with purple/blue discoloration and blanching on pressure	Inspiratory stridor or sighs
Emotional incontinence (crying without sadness or laughing without mirth)	Severe dysphonia, dysarthria, and/or dysarthria
	Raynaud's phenomenon in hands and feet, predominantly

*, ** Features presented at the first and second evaluation, respectively.

In Video 13b, patient demonstrates early dystonic posturing in his left hand. Some of the examination "red flags" are illustrated in Video 13d (adapted from Köllensperger et al.[4]).

Other atypical features that should raise the diagnostic suspicion for MSA are listed in Table 3.1.[4] Besides an impaired tandem gait, which could have been considered an atypical finding for PD at the earliest evaluation session,[5] orofacial dyskinesias and postural instability within 3 years were the first decidedly atypical features in this case. Dystonic posturing of the left hand began to develop at the second evaluation. Selected examples of these "red flags" are contained within Video 13d.

Diagnosis: Multiple system atrophy, parkinsonian type

Tip: *When present, L-dopa-induced dyskinesias in MSA often involve the oromandibular region.*

Case 14: Intermittent "risus sardonicus" in a young man

Case: This previously healthy 20-year-old man progressively developed slurred speech, drooling, and bilateral hand tremor over the 10 months preceding this evaluation. The tremor was first noticed while writing. His performance in college had also deteriorated. A facial expression that was reminiscent of the case just discussed above was noted during the interview (Video 14a).

Should the facial appearance have helped to focus the examination?

Indeed, this is the characteristic facial dystonia of Wilson's disease, giving the "risus sardonicus" appearance to the perioral region. One could describe this as a "smirk" because of the upward pull of the upper lip, a "smile evoking insolence, scorn, or offensive smugness," as per Wikipedia. Although intermittent in this case, it may persist in those who may go untreated for a longer time (Video 14b). The next highest-yield examination step is to look for the one place where copper can be visible, at the junction between the cornea and sclera, on the edge of the iris. This brown corneal halo, the Kayser-Fleischer ring, was confirmed in this patient by slit-lamp examination. Incidentally, copper may also be deposited in the lens capsule causing "sunflower cataracts."

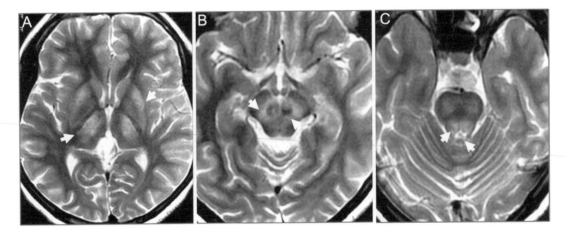

Figure 3.2. Brain T2-weighted axial MRI demonstrates (A) symmetric hyperintense signals in the putamen (left arrow), posterior internal capsule, and thalami (right arrow), (B) "face of the giant panda" in midbrain with high signal in tegmentum and normal red nuclei (arrows), and (C) "face of the panda cub" in pons with hypointensity of central tegmental tracts with hyperintensity of aqueductal opening to fourth ventricle (arrows). Taken with permission from Shivakumar and Thomas.[6]

Could other "faces" (with fewer smirks) have helped in Wilson's disease?

Yes, the faces of the giant panda and its small cub, which can only be recognized with a brain MRI (Figure 3.2).

Are there pitfalls in the laboratory investigations to confirm Wilson's disease?

Yes, low urinary copper and "normal" ceruloplasmin. A reason patients are sent to specialists "for further evaluation of possible Wilson's disease" is because a 24-hour urinary copper was below the normal range. This, in fact, would exclude the diagnosis – though a different diagnosis may still be made (see below). What is paradoxically low in Wilson's disease is the serum copper, since the problem with copper in the body is not of deficiency but of poor distribution because the "distributor" (ceruloplasmin) is in short supply, resulting in low serum copper but high free serum copper. This leads to copper accumulation in the cornea, liver, and the brain. The second laboratory pitfall is "normal" ceruloplasmin. Because it is an acute phase reactant, ceruloplasmin may be elevated into the normal range during inflammatory states. Hence, diagnosis is based on *low* serum copper, *low* serum ceruloplasmin (in the absence of systemic inflammation), but *high* urinary excretion of copper (in the absence of renal failure). Urinary copper above 100 μg/24 hours (1.6 μmol/24 hours) confirms Wilson's disease, and levels above 40 μg/24 hours (0.6 μmol/24 hours) are strongly suggestive of the diagnosis.

When urinary copper is truly low rather than high, where should the problem be?

In the spinal cord. When low copper and low ceruloplasmin combine with *low* urinary copper, the diagnosis is copper deficiency. The clinical presentation is entirely different: a non-compressive myelopathy, closely mimicking subacute combined degeneration due to vitamin B_{12} deficiency.[7] The treatment strategy is based on copper supplementation.[8]

When ceruloplasmin is not just low but absent, does copper accumulate more?

Not copper, but definitely iron. In aceruloplasminemia, iron accumulates diffusely in the basal ganglia, creating a craniofacial dystonia that may be similar in distribution to that seen in Wilson's disease but typically far more severe (as it happens in other 'neurodegenerations with brain iron accumulation' disorders such as PANK2- associated neurodegeneration and neuroferritinopathy). Iron also deposits in the pancreas and retina and leads to diabetes and retinal degeneration. The diagnosis relies on low serum and urine copper, absent ceruloplasmin, low serum iron, and high serum ferritin. Ceruloplasmin is a ferroxidase, essential for mobilizing ferric iron from reticuloendothelial stores into transferrin. The causative ceruloplasmin gene mutations of aceruloplasminemia raise tissue iron but not copper. Excessive iron declares its presence as diffuse *hypo*intensities on the striatum, thalamus, and dentate nucleus on T2-weighted brain MRI (conversely, Wilson's disease manifests *hyper*intensities in the striatum and thalamus on the same MRI sequence). The treatment strategy is based on desferrioxamine, an iron chelating agent. A case previously thought to represent "hypoceruloplasminemia" (ataxia, dysarthria, and hyperreflexia) was indeed reclassified as having Wilson's disease with absent KF rings after genetic testing.[9]

Discussion: Though a diagnosis of Wilson's disease is based on the presence of low serum ceruloplasmin and high 24-hour urinary copper, the sardonic grin of these patients, when present, should help anticipate the laboratory outcome. When abnormally high, the sensitive 24-hour urinary copper (especially if KF rings are present) renders a liver biopsy superfluous.[10] The copper chelators penicillamine and trientine increase urinary excretion of copper, while zinc and tetrathiomolybdate (not widely available) block copper absorption from the intestine.[11] The treating clinician is wise to remember that many patients presenting with neurological symptoms may worsen with penicillamine, which also increases the risk for drug-induced lupus

and may unmask or worsen myasthenia gravis.[12] Trientine produces a rapid negative copper balance whereas zinc's effect in inducing liver metallothionein is slower in sequestering hepatic copper. Zinc has been advocated as the initial treatment of choice in mild to moderate cases and for use during maintenance because of its efficacy and relative lack of toxicity (though at high doses, zinc might induce copper deficiency myelopathy).[7] In patients with associated mild liver failure, a combination of trientine and zinc may be preferred.[13] The appropriate choice of copper-chelation (penicillamine, trientine) or copper-wasting strategies (tetrathiomolybdate, zinc) should transform a smirk into a genuinely beaming grin.

Diagnosis: Wilson's disease

Tip: *Spontaneous and action-induced facial dystonia giving a sardonic or "smirky" appearance can be a subtle presentation of Wilson's disease.*

Case 15: Resting and postural tremor: PD or ET?

Case: A 63-year-old man with slowly progressive right-hand tremor for 4 years was evaluated for possible PD. The tremor was present at rest but also interfered with his ability to work as an electrician and carpenter. Over the past 3 months, the tremor had appeared, to a mild extent, in the left hand. He received pramipexole which improved his known restless leg syndrome but it had to be discontinued due to dizziness. The focused review of systems geared for someone suspected of having PD was of questionable assistance. He endorsed some hyposmia, mild urinary urgency, and occasional postural lightheadedness but no constipation, erectile dysfunction, depression, or dream enactment behaviors.

Examination showed mild right-hand tremor at rest, with greater postural tremor, also involving the left hand (Video 15a). There was no latency between assumption of outstretched posture and initiation of the tremor. The action tremor was of approximately equal magnitude to the postural tremor. Rapid alternating movements were somewhat slow but no fatiguing occurred.

What important piece of history could further help answer the PD-vs-ET dilemma?

After 4 years of tremor, handwriting should typically be affected. In PD, one expects smaller handwriting the longer individuals write. In ET, the size of handwritten notes may not change but the quality is often chaotic. This man's handwriting was described as "large and messy." This historical piece of information is as valuable during a telephone consultation as witnessing the arm swinging in the hall during a "curbside consult." This patient, in fact, showed greater arm swinging in the right, more affected hand, compared to the less affected one (see last segment of Video 15a). Hence, the bulk of the evidence strongly favored essential tremor. He experienced marked improvement within 2 weeks of reaching a propranolol dose of 20 mg/day (Video 15b).

Discussion: Although advanced ET patients can have resting tremor, it is likely that this patient was not truly at rest when the first video segment was taken. His may very well have been a pseudo-rest tremor. In addition to this "rest" component, the tremor was unilateral at onset. These two elements were rightly interpreted as possibly representing PD. Even if the tremor was truly present at rest, it should be born in mind that rest tremor can be part of the phenotypic spectrum of ET in 1 out of 5 patients, typically associated with more severe and longer-lasting disease, often with larger amplitude and lower frequency tremor.[14] Further, a rest tremor may not necessarily reflect underlying Lewy body pathology in the substantia nigra.[15] Similarly, unilateral tremor may occur in almost 5% of ET patients for up to 5 years from symptom onset.[16] Overall, the examination features and robust and sustained response to propranolol strongly support the clinical diagnosis of ET.[17]

In situations of long-standing tremor, the possibility of comorbid ET and PD should be born in

mind and a trial with L-dopa worth considering. A history of action-induced tremor (spilling beans, jerky handwriting), which would suggest ET, is not exclusionary of PD if (1) the resting component of such tremor exacerbates with activating maneuvers, (2) there is fatiguing on finger tapping, (3) the tremor becomes more visible during walking on the side with reduced arm swinging, and (4) the patient has noted leg tremor ipsilateral to the arm tremor or leg tremor becomes apparent during the course of the examination (Video 15c). In these cases, an excellent response to L-dopa is reassuring (Video 15d).

Diagnosis: Essential tremor

Tip: *Unilaterality or marked asymmetry of tremor and a resting component do not necessarily exclude a diagnosis of ET. Tremor at "rest" may actually represent posture holding when the limbs are insufficiently relaxed.*

Case 16: Restlessness of some sort

Case: This 27-year-old woman was referred to our center for evaluation of worsening "hyperactivity" over the prior 12 months. She had been "fidgety" and feeling more "full of energy" than usual. Lately, she felt like having racing thoughts and "thinking about thinking" (Video 16a). She had been more obsessive about checking that door knobs were locked. She reported no history of vocal or motor tics. She had taken oral contraceptives since the age of 16 years.

How do mental and motor tasks help define the phenotype?

Except for the suppressable tics, mental and selected motor tasks are best at bringing on the two core hyperkinetic disorders underlying "restlessness," chorea and myoclonus. This patient showed distal "piano-playing" finger movements and rapid jerks of her trunk largely when performing arithmetic tests with her eyes closed. She would otherwise mask her restlessness within other voluntary or semi-voluntary activities. Importantly, writing did not accentuate any movements. Observing patients during writing

Table 3.2. Three main etiologic categories of non-degenerative chorea in a young woman

1. Iatrogenic	2. Endocrine/immunologic	3. Infections/immunologic*
Oral contraceptives	Hyperthyroidism	Antiphospholipid antibody syndrome
Cocaine	Hyperglycemia	Systemic lupus erythematosus
Anticonvulsants	Hypoparathyroidism	Lyme disease
Antidepressants	Polycythemia rubra vera	AIDS (especially PML)
Neuroleptics		Sydenham's disease
Stimulants		
L-dopa		

* Some of these may be progressive.

AIDS: acquired immune deficiency syndrome; PML: progressive multifocal leukoencephalopathy.

is critical since this may be the only task during which myoclonic jerks can appear in the shoulder girdle and neck regions in myoclonus dystonia (M-D)[18] (Video 16b). Finally, there were no brief stereotypic, patterned movements *between* (rather than *within*) voluntary movements to suggest tics. Hence, the overarching phenotype in this case is chorea, mild, apparently not progressive. The rest of the neurological examination was normal.

How does one unravel the etiology of mild chorea in a young woman?

Ascertaining the phenotype of "restlessness" as mild chorea in young adulthood is critical in considering the evaluation for the three main categories of disorders that may explain it: drug-induced, endocrine/immunologic, and infections (Table 3.2).[19] The plan of attack is, thus, as follows. First, a thorough review of drug exposures. Oral contraceptives and cocaine are the usual suspects at this age. If no drugs can account for the chorea, the next step is to delve into the endocrine/immunologic work up. A high-yield set of investigations includes a search for hyperthyroidism, hyperglycemia, hypoparathyroidism, and polycythemia vera,[20] followed by antiphospholipid antibody syndrome and lupus.[21] A neuroimaging study may be helpful in determining the etiology by ascertaining the extent and pattern of parenchymal involvement (e.g., head CT to examine for calcium deposition in the basal ganglia and cerebellum in the setting of hypoparathyroidism, or brain MRI to determine extent of microangiopathic changes in the antiphospholipid antibody syndrome).

After the work up suggested above turned unrevealing, oral contraceptives were discontinued to no avail. Anti-streptolysin O (ASO) antibodies (395 IU/mL) and anti-DNAse B titers were elevated (960 Todd units/mL [normal, < 85]). More than 90% of streptococcal infections can be identified with the combination of abnormal ASO and anti-DNAse B titers. Culture for group A β-hemolytic streptococcal (GABHS) infection in the throat was positive. The diagnosis of Sydenham's disease was made. A 10-day course of penicillin-V 500 mg three times daily was initiated, with subsequent resolution of symptoms.

Discussion: Sydenham's disease (SD) can complicate a GABHS infection presumably because of molecular mimicry. Although more common in children, SD can also be a cause of "restlessness" (mild chorea or myoclonus) in adolescents and young adults. Clinical clues include difficulty with fine motor tasks, inattention, anxiety, and obsessive compulsive behaviors.[22] Two main pitfalls need to be avoided in its management: First, as a form of rheumatic fever, SD may also be associated with carditis (valvulopathy) and arthritis. The treating clinician should not forget to screen for these comorbidities. Second, SD increases the susceptibility to developing other later-onset choreas, such as those induced by oral contraceptives, estrogen-containing creams, and pregnancy (chorea gravidarum). The chorea of oral contraceptives begins months after drug initiation and ends within weeks of withdrawal.[23] This particular patient should be counseled that the future use of oral contraceptives and pregnancy will need neurological monitoring due to the increased risk of chorea recurrence. A brief course with benzodiazepines, valproic acid, or a neuroleptic to treat chorea directly is rarely necessary. Anticholinergic agents should certainly not be used. Secondary prevention with penicillin or comparable antibiotic, in patients younger than 21 years, reduces the risk of future GABHS infections causing permanent cardiac valvulopathy.

One final word: if the "restlessness of some sort" were to have been present since childhood, and reported in other members of the family, a genetic disorder might have been considered: benign hereditary chorea (BHC). BHC is a non-progressive autosomal dominant chorea due to mutations in the *TITF-1* gene on chromosome 14q. An early history of congenital hypothyroidism and respiratory distress is supportive of this diagnosis.

Diagnosis: Sydenham's disease

Tip: *the treatable chorea of Sydenham's disease may be masked as "restlessness" and can be easily missed or overlooked in young adults, when it is less common than in childhood.*

Case 17: Mild orofacial dyskinesias in parkinsonism

Case: This 58-year-old man complained of slowness, poor dexterity, and hand tremor over a period of 2 years. Examination showed hypomimia, bilateral postural tremor of the hands, bradykinesia, and mild rigidity. More recently, his spouse had noted movements around the nose and lips about which he was unaware (Video 17a).

How can the facial movements be described?

With animal analogies: a cow and a rabbit. A cow is a *ruminant* that repetitively brings up and chews previously swallowed food, grass or hay, to aid in its digestion. A rabbit wiggles its nose to constantly monitor the environment for danger, and splits its upper lip to moisturize the air and improve the ability to pick up scents. The movements in this man can be said to have a mixture of *rumination* and nose wiggling. The full-blown "rabbit syndrome,"[24] which reflects a more rhythmic abnormality than what was appreciated in this case (Video 17b), was absent. In this case, the overarching phenomenology was more akin to *rumination*, the subtle orofacial dyskinesia suggestive of a tardive complication and strongly supporting the suspicion that the associated parkinsonism may have been induced by a neuroleptic.

How does the phenomenological characterization help in managing this man?

Whereas the "rabbit syndrome" does not fully help define the underlying etiology, and can be present in drug-induced and idiopathic parkinsonism, the "ruminating" orofacial dyskinesia belongs to the spectrum of tardive dyskinesia. Hence, a careful search for neuroleptic exposure becomes mandatory in this man. Indeed, for several years, he was on treatment with metoclopramide, 10 mg three times per day for chronic nausea due to gastroesophageal reflux disease. A recommendation was made to discontinue this neuroleptic medication and to consider a safer anti-nausea strategy.

Discussion: Metoclopramide and prochlorperazine are two commonly used antiemetics, often unsuspected sources of parkinsonism when compared to antipsychotics. These antiemetics, like most antipsychotics, have dopamine receptor blocking properties (for which they are termed *neuroleptics*) and are capable of inducing parkinsonism as well as a variety of other movement disorders. Organized according to the order of appearance after drug initiation, the range of neuroleptic-induced movement disorders includes acute dystonic reactions, acute akathisia, parkinsonism, neuroleptic malignant syndrome, and tardive syndromes (including tardive dyskinesia, dystonia, tics, and akathisia).[25] It is not uncommon for two or more drug-induced movement disorders to occur simultaneously in the same patient, such as parkinsonism and the "ruminating" tardive dyskinesia of this case.[26] The more common phenotype of tardive dyskinesia, however, is the buccolinguomasticatory form, in which, beyond the purposeless chewing (or rumination), the tongue is involved, with repetitive twisting and protrusion.[27] Movements may persist or worsen over time, despite, or sometimes because of, drug withdrawal. The blockade of striatal D2 receptors is believed to account for acute dystonic reactions and especially drug-induced parkinsonism. Akathisia and neuroleptic malignant syndrome are likely due to more widespread dopamine antagonistic effects. The pathogenesis of tardive dyskinesia, which typically requires longer-term neuroleptic use, is not well understood but probably involves factors distinct from pure D2 receptor blockade.

Although drug-induced *parkinsonism* can be indistinguishable from PD, two features in this case were highly suggestive of an iatrogenic problem: an exclusively postural component of the tremor and the presence of the ruminating orofacial dyskinesia. Metoclopramide is more likely to cause parkinsonism among patients with renal failure and dose reduction or elimination is prudent in this setting.[28] Patients with disabling iatrogenic parkinsonism may not improve sufficiently from withdrawal of the offending neuroleptic and temporary symptomatic treatment with L-dopa or a dopamine agonist may be necessary. More persistent symptoms suggest the possibility of an underlying primary parkinsonian disorder (possibly occult at the time of drug initiation) that could have predisposed the patient to this complication. To avoid the parkinsonism due to neuroleptic-type antiemetics, the drugs of choice for antiemetic control and upper gastrointestinal tract motility disorders, especially in the elderly, are domperidone, a peripheral dopamine antagonist, or ondansetron, a selective serotonin 5-HT$_3$ receptor antagonist.[29]

Diagnosis: metoclopramide-induced parkinsonism and tardive dyskinesia

Tip: *Review the current and past drug lists of patients with parkinsonism especially in the presence of any orofacial dyskinesias, with or without tongue involvement.*

Case 18: Speech arrests in Parkinson's disease

Case: This 73-year-old woman developed left arm resting tremor, hypophonia, and micrographia, leading to the diagnosis of Parkinson's disease after 2 years from symptom onset. She exhibited an excellent response to L-dopa. Three years after initiation of treatment, she developed motor complications with wearing off and peak-dose, L-dopa-induced dyskinesias, which were controlled by modestly lowering the dose of L-dopa and introducing amantadine. Within the next year, she started to notice some speech problems, with frequent arrests, impairing her ability to communicate (Video 18a).

Which are the subtle findings that hold the key to the problem?

The very subtle myoclonic facial movements present during speech, and in the hands when holding the arms outstretched. Myoclonus is not a feature of uncomplicated PD. Hence, this development implies that we are not dealing with PD, that dementia has been superimposed, or that an "extrinsic" variable (e.g., a drug or drugs) is at play. Given a seven-year course without (other) unusual motor features or objective deterioration of cognitive function, an atypical parkinsonism or PD dementia seem improbable. The speech abnormality is unlike that of MSA where myoclonus may more commonly be seen in the outstretched hands. A more reasonable possibility, easier to evaluate, is that she has developed another complication of her treatment regimen. Both L-dopa and amantadine can induce myoclonus, but the nature of this complication differs. L-dopa rarely causes myoclonus and a tighter relationship with each dosing cycle may occur. Amantadine-induced myoclonus typically affects the speech, as seen in this patient.

Shall we first reduce or discontinue amantadine to test the hypothesis?

Indeed, since she is benefiting most from L-dopa. After amantadine 300 mg/day was discontinued, the speech impairment and subtle myoclonic movements disappeared. However, L-dopa-induced dyskinesias worsened. Amantadine was reintroduced at 100 mg. Dyskinesias remained tolerable and neither speech arrests nor myoclonic movements recurred (Video 18b).

Discussion: The subtle hand and finger jerks of this case were repetitive but arrhythmic and could not have been categorized as tremor. Instead, they are best described as fine myoclonic individual finger jerks seen in the outstretched hands ("polyminimyoclonus"), much as occurs in MSA.[30] The speech arrests were likely due to action-induced myoclonic activity in the tongue and oral muscles, as previously described,[31] since they disappeared along with the myoclonus elsewhere after amantadine was reduced. Incidentally, she did not appear to have been aware of her myoclonic hand movements but her related speech impairment brought them to our attention.

In PD, myoclonus can be a complication of L-dopa and amantadine. The multifocal action-induced or spontaneous myoclonus related to L-dopa is observed during the onset-of-dose dyskinesia.[32] Since it disappears partially or completely once optimal clinical efficacy is achieved, this complication corresponds to a state of intermediate dopaminergic stimulation.[33] As the timing of this patient's speech impairment was not clearly related to the dose cycles, the L-dopa theory does not hold water. Amantadine, on the other hand, is typically associated with multifocal myoclonus of the limbs and orofacial region, and disappears when treatment is stopped.[31;34] Involvement of speech may be a more common iatrogenic phenomenon than usually recognized.[35] This complication may be expected with greater frequency among those with associated renal dysfunction because approximately 90% of the oral dose of amantadine is excreted in the urine and little amantadine can be removed by hemodialysis.[36] Amantadine-induced myoclonus might result from an increased release of serotonin because amantadine can inhibit serotonin reuptake in presynaptic neurons.

Diagnosis: Amantadine-induced orofacial and limb myoclonus in PD

Tip: *Myoclonic activity in Parkinson's disease is most commonly iatrogenic in the absence of dementia. A reduction or discontinuation of amantadine resolves the problem.*

REFERENCES

1. Wenning GK, Geser F, Poewe W. The 'risus sardonicus' of multiple system atrophy. *Mov Disord* 2003;**18**(10):1211.

2. Boesch SM, Wenning GK, Ransmayr G, et al. Dystonia in multiple system atrophy. *J Neurol Neurosurg Psychiatry* 2002;**72**(3):300–303.

3. Delfs JM, Kelley AE. The role of D1 and D2 dopamine receptors in oral stereotypy induced by dopaminergic stimulation of the ventrolateral striatum. *Neuroscience* 1990;**39**(1):59–67.

4. Kollensperger M, Geser F, Seppi K, et al. Red flags for multiple system atrophy. *Mov Disord* 2008;**23**(8):1093–1099.

5. Abdo WF, Borm GF, Munneke M, et al. Ten steps to identify atypical parkinsonism. *J Neurol Neurosurg Psychiatry* 2006;**77**(12):1367–1369.

6. Shivakumar R, Thomas SV. Teaching NeuroImages: face of the giant panda and her cub: MRI correlates of Wilson disease. *Neurology* 2009;**72**(11):e50.

7. Kumar N, Gross JB, Jr., Ahlskog JE. Copper deficiency myelopathy produces a clinical picture like subacute combined degeneration. *Neurology* 2004;**63**(1):33–39.

8. Kumar N, Butz JA, Burritt MF. Clinical significance of the laboratory determination of low serum copper in adults. *Clin Chem Lab Med* 2007;**45**(10):1402–1410.

9. Mehta SH, Parekh SM, Prakash R, et al. Predominant ataxia, low ceruloplasmin, and absent K-F rings: hypoceruloplasminemia or Wilson's disease. *Mov Disord* 2010;**25**(13):2260–2261.

10. Walshe JM. Monitoring copper in Wilson's disease. *Adv Clin Chem* 2010;**50**:151–163.

11. Brewer GJ. The use of copper-lowering therapy with tetrathiomolybdate in medicine. *Expert Opin Investig Drugs* 2009;**18**(1):89–97.

12. Brewer GJ. Neurologically presenting Wilson's disease: epidemiology, pathophysiology and treatment. *CNS Drugs* 2005;**19**(3):185–192.

13. Brewer GJ. Practical recommendations and new therapies for Wilson's disease. *Drugs* 1995;**50**(2):240–249.

14. Cohen O, Pullman S, Jurewicz E, et al. Rest tremor in patients with essential tremor: prevalence, clinical correlates, and electrophysiologic characteristics. *Arch Neurol* 2003;**60**(3):405–410.

15. Louis ED, Asabere N, Agnew A, et al. Rest tremor in advanced essential tremor: a post-mortem study of nine cases. *J Neurol Neurosurg Psychiatry* 2011;**82**:261–265.

16. Phibbs F, Fang JY, Cooper MK, et al. Prevalence of unilateral tremor in autosomal dominant essential tremor. *Mov Disord* 2009;**24**(1):108–111.

17. Louis ED. Essential tremor. *Lancet Neurol* 2005;**4**(2):100–110.

18. Kinugawa K, Vidailhet M, Clot F, et al. Myoclonus-dystonia: an update. *Mov Disord* 2009;**24**(4):479–489.

19. Higgins DS, Jr. Chorea and its disorders. *Neurol Clin* 2001;**19**(3):707–722, vii.

20. Mas JL, Gueguen B, Bouche P, et al. Chorea and polycythaemia. *J Neurol* 1985;**232**(3):169–171.

21. Wild EJ, Tabrizi SJ. The differential diagnosis of chorea. *Pract Neurol* 2007;**7**(6):360–373.

22. Gilbert DL. Acute and chronic chorea in childhood. *Semin Pediatr Neurol* 2009;**16**(2):71–76.

23. Wadlington WB, Erlendson IW, Burr IM. Chorea associated with the use of oral contraceptives: report of a case and review of the literature. *Clin Pediatr (Phila)* 1981;**20**(12):804–806.

24. Wada Y, Yamaguchi N. The rabbit syndrome and anti-parkinsonian medication in schizophrenic patients. *Neuropsychobiology* 1992;**25**(3):149–152.

25. Espay AJ. Toxic movement disorders: the approach to the patient with a movement disorder of toxic origin. In: Dobbs M, ed. *Clinical Neurotoxicology*. Amsterdam, The Netherlands: Elsevier, 2009;115–130.

26. Grimes JD. Parkinsonism and tardive dyskinesia associated with long-term metoclopramide therapy. *N Engl J Med* 1981;**305**(23):1417.

27. Margolese HC, Chouinard G, Kolivakis TT, et al. Tardive dyskinesia in the era of typical and atypical antipsychotics. Part 2: Incidence and management strategies in patients with schizophrenia. *Can J Psychiatry* 2005;**50**(11):703–714.

28. Sethi KD, Patel B, Meador KJ. Metoclopramide-induced parkinsonism. *South Med J* 1989;**82**(12):1581–1582.

29. Wilde MI, Markham A. Ondansetron: a review of its pharmacology and preliminary clinical findings in novel applications. *Drugs* 1996;**52**(5):773–794.

30. Abdo WF, van de Warrenburg BP, Burn DJ, et al. The clinical approach to movement disorders. *Nat Rev Neurol* 2010;**6**(1):29–37.

31. Matsunaga K, Uozumi T, Qingrui L, et al. Amantadine-induced cortical myoclonus. *Neurology* 2001;**56**(2):279–280.

32. Defebvre L. Myoclonus and extrapyramidal diseases. *Neurophysiol Clin* 2006;**36**(5–6):319–325.

33. Shafiq M, Lang AE. Myoclonus in parkinsonian disorders. *Adv Neurol* 2002;**89**:77–83.

34. Pfeiffer RF. Amantadine-induced "vocal" myoclonus. *Mov Disord* 1996;**11**(1):104–106.

35. Gupta A, Lang AE. Drug-induced cranial myoclonus. *Mov Disord* 2010;**25**(13):2264–2265.

36. Aoki FY, Sitar DS. Clinical pharmacokinetics of amantadine hydrochloride. *Clin Pharmacokinet* 1988;**14**(1):35–51.

4

When movement disorders are difficult to characterize

Case 19: An unusual tremor for PD

Case: This 54-year-old woman had difficulties with handwriting dating back 7 years ago. She described her handwriting as "messy." Over time, she developed sore muscles, tiredness, leg cramps, arm cramps, and back cramps. About 4 years ago, she developed a tremor in her right hand, mostly present while feeding and performing other tasks, but absent at rest. She denied hyposmia or constipation. She was diagnosed with PD and offered enrollment into a clinical trial of a putative neuroprotective agent.

What elements from this history argue against the diagnosis of PD?

Several: (1) "messy" rather than small handwriting; (2) cramps everywhere rather than restricted to the thighs or calves; (3) action rather than resting tremor; and (4) absence of historical support for major non-motor symptoms of PD, hyposmia and constipation. Before examining her, our skepticism kicked into high gear.

What elements of the examination reinforce our skepticism?

The examination demonstrated no resting tremor. Instead, there was a jerky postural one that modestly worsened over 2 years (Video 19). Assessment of rapid alternating movements demonstrated no decrement or fatiguing. The hands showed subtle finger posturing and arrhythmic jerking when the arms were held outstretched. Handwriting was not micrographic. The patient was informed of the revised diagnosis and asked to discontinue her participation in the clinical trial. A β-CIT SPECT scan was normal. Two years later and still without treatment there was milder worsening of her jerky tremor but no resting component or any other symptoms. Arm swing remained unimpaired.

Discussion: Tremor and bradykinesia are arguably the most common reasons for the misdiagnosis of PD. Tremor usually predominates at rest, although some patients only have a positional and action tremor. Here, other features including bradykinesia and rigidity are mandatory. Bradykinesia should be accompanied by decrement and fatiguing if PD is the correct pathology. Bradykinesia in the pseudo-parkinsonism of cerebellar or dystonic disorders is not associated with decrement or fatiguing.[1] This patient's overall diagnostic flavor was that of dystonia, rather than a hypokinetic disorder.[2] Dystonic tremor, abnormal posturing, and lack of true bradykinesia suggested the diagnosis of dystonia. The negative scan established the otherwise non-committal research-based label of "Scans Without Evidence of Dopaminergic Deficits" or SWEDDs.[3] Dystonic tremor is an important cause of SWEDDs and must be recognized to minimize the ~15% of patients admitted into PD clinical trials who have normal nigrostriatal uptake of presynaptic ligands and, presumably, no true PD. Although patients with SWEDDs may present with a more typical PD-like picture, consisting of an asymmetric resting hand tremor, even with a re-emergent component on posture, and impaired arm swing, their rapid alternating movements never exhibit the classical decrement or fatiguing of true bradykinesia.[4] Other features suggesting dystonia in SWEDDs are "thumb extension" tremor, task- or position-specific tremor, head tremor, dystonic voice, and no progression into features other than tremor and dystonia.[4]

Diagnosis: Dystonia (SWEDDs)

Tip: *Jerky, irregular resting tremor is a manifestation of dystonia that may be incorrectly interpreted as representing PD. Dystonic tremor may account for a large proportion of patients with SWEDDs.*

Case 20: Another unusual tremor for PD

Case: An 81-year-old man first noticed an abnormality 3 years prior to his first evaluation with us when he "lost use of my left arm." The first problem was tremor and posturing but progressively he noticed that the arm was not moving at will. He observed that it would rise for no apparent reason. Over time, he noted that the left leg became weak and uncoordinated. Six months prior to this assessment he needed a walker and, shortly thereafter, a wheelchair. His speech volume had softened and his swallowing was slow, requiring him to frequently clear his throat.

What elements from this history argue against the diagnosis of PD?

The two most powerful are the introductory symptom, "losing" the use of an arm, and the timeline. Requiring assistance with walking within 3 years from the onset of symptoms is not within the plausible rate of progression for PD. The episodes of arm levitation described represent another major red flag. Arm levitation may be the earliest stage of the alien limb syndrome, a sign of parieto-occipital dysfunction, squarely pointing in the direction of corticobasal syndrome (CBS).

Can the examination help predict the etiology of this suspected corticobasal syndrome?

The only element of the examination that is relatively etiology-specific is tremor. This patient showed a high-frequency, high-amplitude unilateral tremor, occurring intermittently at rest and on posture (Video 20a). In an autopsy study of patients with CBS, such tremor was present in three quarters of 16 patients with pathology-proven corticobasal degeneration (CBD) but in no cases with CBS due to AD,[5] in whom myoclonus was more common (Video 20b). The patient also demonstrated a markedly asymmetric parkinsonism with rigidity and dystonia, sensory extinction and agraphesthesia, as well as a hemiparetic gait, though these elements do not help predict pathology. Cognitive impairment by bedside screening was demonstrated to be mild to moderate (MMSE = 21/30; Frontal Assessment Battery = 16/18; abnormal clock drawing). His brain MRI showed moderate atrophy in the parietal and, to a lesser extent, temporal lobes, greater in the right hemisphere. There was mild ex-vacuo enlargement of the occipital horn of the right lateral ventricle.

Discussion: A rapidly progressive and profoundly asymmetric akinetic-rigid syndrome with severe arm dystonia and rigidity, tremor, and historic evidence of arm levitation (early alien limb syndrome) in the setting of cortical sensory loss in the left arm suggest the presence of CBS. Of the clinical features associated with CBS, tremor is most helpful as it most often correlates with CBD as the underlying pathology (Table 4.1).[5] The other features, including ideomotor and limb kinetic apraxia (confirmed before dystonia and rigidity become severe) and action or stimulus-sensitive myoclonus, have been reported in a range of disorders including vascular disease, AD, PSP, CJD, DLB, and FLTD. In fact, most cases of CBS are due to PSP rather than CBD pathology. These cases of CBS-PSP have delayed onset of vertical supra-nuclear gaze palsy (> 3 years after onset of first symptom) and rarely have predominant downgaze abnormalities.[6]

Table 4.1. Clinical features associated with CBD and AD as the pathology of CBS

More common in CBD	Same in CBD and AD	More common in AD
Older age (60s)	Ideomotor limb apraxia	Younger age (50s)
Tremor	Alien limb syndrome	No tremor
Apraxia of speech*	Rigidity and dystonia	Myoclonus
	Cortical sensory loss	
	Memory impairment	
From a memory-clinic perspective**		
Non-fluent aphasia		Initial episodic memory
Oculomotor apraxia		
Oculo-buccal facial apraxia		
Frontal utilization behavior		

* Apraxia of speech is a motor disorder with the features of hesitancy, effortfulness with articulatory groping, phonetic errors, and dysprosody, which is often part of the progressive non-fluent aphasia form of frontotemporal dementia and localizes to the left posterior inferior frontal lobe atrophy. This is in contrast with orofacial apraxia which is due to left middle frontal, premotor, and supplementary motor cortical atrophy; and limb apraxia, due to left inferior parietal lobe atrophy.[8]

** CBD patients do not exhibit early episodic memory complaints. Conversely, none of those with CBS due to AD have frontal lobe behavioral changes. Compared with AD, CBD patients more commonly show apathy, irritability, socially inappropriate disinhibited behavior, emotional lability, stereotypic behavior, and lack of insight. Besides CBS, other focal presentations of AD are posterior cortical atrophy and the progressive non-fluent aphasia variant of FTD, but rarely semantic dementia or the behavioral variant of FTD.[9] Adapted from Hu et al.[5] and Shelley et al.[10]

The presence of an alien limb does not help in sorting out the CBD vs. AD dilemma. The "frontal variant" alien-like behavior most closely resembles the exploratory reaching, grasping, and other purposeful movements, and may be more commonly seen as a severe form of grasp reflex in the setting of anteromedial frontal lobe degeneration. The "frontal" alien hand cannot release an object from grasp without the contralateral hand "peeling" the fingers away from the grasped object. The "posterior variant" of alien limb, which may be more frequently described in CBD and AD, demonstrates an "instinctive avoidance reaction," in which the digits extend and the hand pulls away from approaching objects. This useless or "avoidant" hand, if otherwise quiet or myoclonic, most likely reflects AD pathology; if associated with tremor, it most likely indicates CBD pathology. Whereas both frontal and posterior alien limb variants can occur in CBD, the frontal variant also could be part of FTLD and the posterior variant is also seen in AD.

Patterns of atrophy on brain MRI can be helpful in distinguishing CBS due to FTLD (frontotemporal), from CBS due to AD (temporoparietal) (Figure 4.1, from Case 20b), or due to CBD or PSP (supplemental motor area).[7]

Diagnosis: Corticobasal syndrome due to pathology-proven corticobasal degeneration.

Tip: *A high-frequency resting and postural tremor in a markedly asymmetric corticobasal syndrome strongly suggests the pathology of CBD. CBS due to AD tends to occur at a younger age than in CBD and is more likely to be associated with myoclonus (or no associated movements) rather than tremor in the more affected, dystonic arm.*

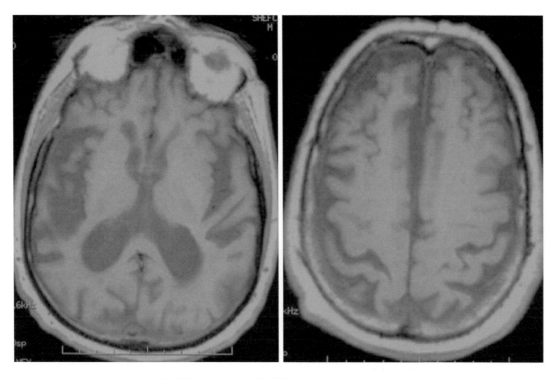

Figure 4.1. Brain T1-weighted axial MRI in a patient with CBS due to AD pathology (Case 20b). The images demonstrate greater temporal than parietal atrophy, with relatively less atrophy in the frontal region.

Case 21: A "dirty essential tremor"

Case: This 39-year-old physician became aware of bilateral hand tremor while dissecting animals in junior college. The tremor was noted only during activities and progressed over several years to affect his ability to drink from a cup and use a spoon or fork. He would often spill beverages and become embarrassed about the possibility of exposing his clumsiness to public scrutiny. He used an electrical razor with both hands and had difficulty with buttoning his shirt. Holding weights worsened his tremor. His handwriting became sloppy but not micrographic. Alcohol had no effect on the tremor although he never drank in excess of two glasses of wine at a single sitting. For about 10 years he had been on treatment with nortriptyline and lamotrigine to address anxiety and depression. His presumed essential tremor benefited modestly

from propranolol but he was switched to pindolol because of worsening depression, which forced him to relinquish his practice. Of interest, sodium oxybate (Xyram), which was prescribed for him in combination with eszopiclone (Lunesta) for insomnia, improved his tremor modestly. Examination showed a high-frequency, low-amplitude postural tremor, with slight worsening during action (Video 21).

Why is the tremor difficult to characterize?

His tremor contained elements of several tremor disorders. Its low amplitude and high frequency was more in keeping with metabolic, iatrogenic, and enhanced physiologic tremor. The increase in amplitude with action is typical of essential and cerebellar tremors.[11] The intermittent jerking might even suggest a dystonic or myoclonic component. The effect of weight on tremor as volunteered by the patient can be helpful. Weight loading decreases tremor amplitude in essential tremor but increases it in enhanced physiologic tremor[12] as well as psychogenic tremor. Thus, this "dirty" tremor was not easily pigeonholed into a single tremor category.

Could his drug regimen be muddying the waters, blurring the phenomenology?

This patient was not on two, but on three tremorogenic drugs: nortriptyline, lamotrigine, and pindolol. Pindolol is often used by psychiatrists as an augmentation strategy for treatment-refractory depression. Furthermore, as a member of the beta-blocker family of drugs, its introduction was mistakenly believed to be potentially helpful in carrying on with the benefits yielded earlier by propranolol, while avoiding its depressant effects. This was not to be. Pindolol is the only tremor-inducing beta-blocker. Its discontinuation from this patient's regimen brought partial but meaningful attenuation of his tremor. Removing nortriptyline considered as the next management step was not deemed necessary.

Discussion: Relatively symmetric, small-amplitude, high-frequency postural tremor tends most commonly to be iatrogenic when occurring first in adults. At a younger age, in the absence of drug exposures, enhanced physiologic tremor shares the same phenotype. The three drugs used to address this patient's anxiety and depression were tremorogenic. Nortriptyline and lamotrigine are common culprits. Other tremor-causing drugs prescribed by psychiatrists include other antidepressants (SSRIs), lithium, valproic acid, carbamazepine, and neuroleptics.[13] The tremor penalty for pindolol is poorly known among psychiatrists and perhaps even less so among neurologists, as beta-blockers are believed to suppress tremors as a class. Pindolol's unique partial β-adrenergic agonist activity leads to what might be seen as paradoxical appearance of tremor.[14] Hence, pindolol is the exception to the rule that all beta-blockers with sufficient CNS-penetration have anti-tremor action. When a drug-induced tremor appears, discontinuing the offending agent(s) is indicated. If such action for

a disabling tremor would greatly jeopardize the psychiatric control in the judgment of the collaborating psychiatrist, possible pharmacological strategies include propranolol, primidone, gabapentin, topiramate, and benzodiazepines.[15]

Diagnosis: iatrogenic tremor, with large effect from pindolol

Tip: *Small-amplitude, high-frequency postural and kinetic tremor is most often drug induced, especially if symmetric. Pindolol is the only beta-blocker associated with tremor worsening.*

Case 22: Is it a mixed movement disorder or a "twitch"?

Case: This 23-year-old woman with previous history of lupus, diagnosed at the age of 21, reported the onset of left thumb shaking at the age of 16 years, mostly at rest but also present during posture holding. Although the shaking remained most visible in the left hand, she also noticed right-hand "tremor" and "twitching" of the thighs. The abnormal movements had progressed over the last 2 years, consistently worse toward the end of the day. Handwriting was associated with cramping of the right thumb. The key piece of information is visual, as the rest of the neurological exam was normal (Video 22a).

Can the movements be characterized?

The finger movements were difficult to characterize. Though at first blush one may have called them "tremulous," the movements were arrhythmic. Their amplitude varied from barely noticeable to wider jerks, not influenced by positional changes and approximately the same at rest and on posture. Individual fingers seemed to move asynchronously and had a jerky component, slower than expected for myoclonus and of smaller amplitude than expected for most tremors. There was no posturing of the fingers. Hence, despite its hyperkinetic appearance, the movements did not fit the bill for tremor, dystonia, or myoclonus. "Dystonia," however, was listed as the default diagnosis in the chart of this patient.

What is it when we cannot tell what it is?

When one cannot commit to any of the *central* jerky movements (myoclonus, dystonia, tics), a *peripheral* movement disorder might be considered. The umbrella of peripheral nerve hyperexcitability is generally where cramps and "twitches" belong. An EMG study would therefore be particularly helpful at this point. In this patient, needle EMG over forearm muscles revealed doublets and triplets firing at a frequency of 40 Hz.

The patient developed recurrent episodes of knee pain and finger swelling followed by pain in the tarsal-metatarsal joints when she walked. Her ANA titer was 1:80, speckled pattern. A rheumatology consultation was requested and after a comprehensive set of investigations, she was diagnosed with mixed tissue connective disorder, an autoimmune disorder characterized by features of systemic lupus erythematosus, systemic sclerosis, and polymyositis. She was started on a short course of prednisone, which improved her arthritis and attenuated the movements (Video 22b). The appearance of comorbid facial myokymia further supported the underlying presence of peripheral nerve hyperexcitability as part of her autoimmune disorder.

Discussion: The magnitude of abnormal movements is typically barely sufficient to move a joint in peripheral nerve hyperexcitability, which is defined as muscle overactivity due to spontaneous discharges of lower motor neurons and popularly operationalized as "twitching." The better term for this peripheral movement is neuromyotonia or electric myokymia, which applies to the sustained muscle activity of peripheral nerve origin expressed as visible rippling movements, slower than fasciculations (also referred to as "bag of worms").[16] Electrophysiologically, these consist of spontaneous and EMG needle-induced irregular trains of doublets, triplets, and multiplets firing at a high intraburst frequency (150–300 Hz; neuromyotonic discharges), and at lower frequencies (< 60 Hz; myokymic discharges).[17] Acquired neuromyotonia can occur as an idiopathic autoimmune syndrome or as a paraneoplastic phenomenon (anti-voltage-gated potassium channel [VGKC], without peripheral neuropathy, also known as Isaac's syndrome),[18] and may be associated with other autoimmune disorders (thymoma, vitiligo, myasthenia gravis, Hashimoto's thyroiditis, or penicillamine treatment),[19] or belong to a genetic disorder such as episodic ataxia type 1 or HMSN. If the disease-specific treatment is not associated with adequate improvement of the abnormal movement, one may consider a trial with carbamazepine or phenytoin, which can be effective through their interaction with voltage-gated sodium channels.

A number of "dystonia mimics" (pseudo-dystonia) are listed in Table 4.2.

Diagnosis: Acquired neuromyotonia

Tip: *Peripheral nerve hyperexcitability disorders may be misdiagnosed as tremor, dystonia, or myoclonus but meet criteria for none. Neuromyotonia and myokymia require evaluation for paraneoplastic, autoimmune, and genetic disorders.*

Case 23: "Tipsy"

Case: This 22-year-old woman reported "pinwheel vision" for 2 weeks. It came on acutely while lying in bed and had been constant since. She described it further as "looking through a fan" at people. She also had left frontal headache and photophobia as well as facial congestion with mild rhinorrhea but no fever or chills for about a week prior to the onset of her vision problems. She had an episode of migraine, seizures, and visual field cut for a day about 2.5 years ago. She admitted to using heroin intravenously in the past and occasionally alcohol and marijuana. She had a family history of a "maternally inherited disease."

She admitted to clumsiness but was largely unaware of the movements noted during the interview and examination (Video 23).

Table 4.2. Disorders that mimic but do not represent true dystonia

Disorder	Brief description
Acquired neuromyotonia (Isaacs' syndrome)	Neuromyotonia due to motor nerve fiber hyperexcitability (current case)
Facial pseudodystonia	Ptosis or pseudoptosis, trismus, hemimasticatory spasm, hemifacial spasm, myotonia, tetanic spasms
Epilepsia partialis continua	Cases where tonic contraction of a body part predominates
Sensory ataxia (pseudoathetosis)	Slow writhing movements caused by loss of proprioception
Stiff-person syndrome	Muscular stiffness and gait difficulty with stimulus-sensitive superimposed painful muscle spasms and exaggerated lumbar lordosis
Sandifer syndrome	Head and neck posturing, occasionally with opisthotonos, that occurs during feeding in infants with gastroesophageal reflux often associated with hiatal hernia
Schwartz-Jampel syndrome	Generalized stiffness from myotonia associated with blepharospasm, blepharophimosis, dwarfism, pinched face with low-set ears, joint limitation, contractures, and bone dysplasia
Satoyoshi syndrome	Painful, intermittent muscle spasms, malabsorption, endocrinopathy with amenorrhea, skeletal abnormalities, and alopecia areata

Other conditions include spasticity, contractures, rotational atlanto-axial subluxation, congenital Klippel-Feil anomaly, Chiari malformation, posterior fossa tumor, syringomyelia, trochlear nerve palsy, and vestibular torticollis. Tonic spasm may be listed as mimic but it truly is a form of paroxysmal dystonia, and the most frequent movement disorder in MS, due to lesions located anywhere within the motor path (midbrain, capsule, cervical cord).

Are we again facing a difficult movement characterization?

The examination showed random jerks in the face and some neck and truncal swaying, which appeared choreiform at first glance but more ataxic as the examination progressed. There also was oculomotor apraxia and intermittent large-amplitude saccadic intrusions. Jerks and postural lapses in the right arm suggested positive and negative myoclonus, more apparent when attempting to hold her arms outstretched and perform the finger-to-nose task. Hence what she described as "typsying over" may be decomposed into ataxia, chaotic saccades within the opsoclonic range, and myoclonus. This phenotype fits within the umbrella of opsoclonus-myoclonus-ataxia syndrome (OMAS), with associated simple motor seizures as documented per her admission EEG. An additional finding on her exam was right homonymous hemianopsia.

How does it all fit?

Her family history of maternal transmission, visual problems, and seizures were highly suggestive of a mitochondrial disease. As part of the work up, a brain MRI demonstrated hyperintensity on T2-weighted and FLAIR sequences with correlation in diffusion-weighted but not in apparent diffusion coefficient sequences (Figure 4.2). These findings were highly suggestive of the restricted vasogenic edema of mitochondrial encephalopathy with lactic acidosis and subcortical strokes (MELAS). This diagnosis fit well: she had a stroke-like lesion at a young age, in a classic location for MELAS,[20] and with seizures.

What are we missing?

Although the occipital pattern was compelling for MELAS, the "maternally inherited disease" needed confirmation. In fact, her mother and several other

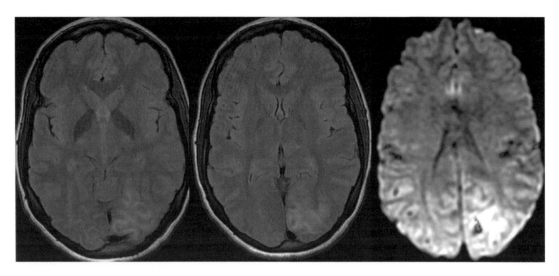

Figure 4.2. FLAIR axial brain MRI (left and center) demonstrates an area of poorly circumscribed hyperintensity in the left occipital region, with corresponding signal abnormality in the diffusion-weighted sequence (right), with normal apparent diffusion coefficient (not shown).

maternal family members had Huntington's disease. In parallel, hospital records from her prior episode of migraine, seizures, and visual field cut 2.5 years ago identified IV heroin as the toxic exposure. The same imaging features so compellingly supportive of MELAS can in fact be seen in heroin addicts.[21] Confronted, the patient admitted to IV use of heroin for 3 days prior to the onset of symptoms. Needless to say, the hunt for mitochondrial mutations, launched before the pieces of this puzzle made sense, was ultimately fruitless.

Discussion: Although the overall phenotype was difficult to characterize, ataxia, a form of oculomotor impairment, and myoclonus, were arguably present in order of declining clarity. The random, high-amplitude, arrhythmic multidirectional conjugate eye movements, sometimes referred to as "chaotic" or "dancing eyes," qualified as opsoclonus. OMAS combines opsoclonus with ataxia and focal or diffuse myoclonus, and is mostly a paraneoplastic disorder in children, typically due to an occult neuroblastoma.[22] In older individuals, it is often a post-infectious disorder due to a variety of infections (e.g., EBV); toxic agents (e.g., lithium)

and malignancies (e.g., lymphoma) have also been reported to cause OMAS, hence the phenotype becomes less specific. In this situation, the imaging abnormality was more helpful – if also incorrectly interpreted at first. The asymmetric occipital lesion was in keeping with the initially suspected diagnosis of MELAS (though the involvement of deep white matter should have been suspect). It was not until further investigative work ruled out a maternally inherited familial disease and documentation of a similar episode in the past proved to have been due to heroin, that the case was recategorized as toxic instead of mitochondrial. Nevertheless, heroin encephalopathy raises lactate in the white matter and responds to antioxidants, suggesting that the common denominator is, still, mitochondrial in nature and that posterior brain regions may be more vulnerable to mitochondrial injuries of genetic or toxic nature. The form of heroin encephalopathy acquired from inhaling its vapors when heated on aluminum foil is known as "chasing the dragon."[23] Severe cases can progress to spastic quadriparesis, pseudobulbar palsy, tremor, chorea, myoclonus, and blindness and may affect, in addition to the white matter of the occipital region, that of the cerebellum, posterior limbs of the internal capsule, splenium of the corpus callosum, medial lemniscus, and lateral brainstem.[23]

Diagnosis: heroin encephalopathy; opsoclonus-myoclonus-ataxia syndrome

Tip: *Toxic exposures (e.g., heroin) may be under-appreciated and go unrecognized behind "educated" explanations (e.g., MELAS) if the story is made to fit. One must make an effort to look for the horse before searching for the zebra.*

Case 24: Slow but not bradykinetic?

Contributed by Dr. Héctor González Usigli, Guadalajara, Jalisco, México

Case: This 54-year-old woman had difficulties with speech, gait, and balance, progressing slowly over the last 4 years. Her main complaint was slowness and clumsiness of her movements and increasing falls. Her examination was remarkable for the presence of spastic dysarthria, bradykinesia, generalized hyperreflexia, and spasticity with Babinski signs and ankle clonus. Her gait was slow and cautious and her postural reflexes severely impaired (Video 24a). Treatment with L-dopa was interpreted as providing modest benefits in postural control and ambulation.

Does she have an atypical parkinsonism?

Her slowness and decreased amplitude of movement prompted an initial diagnosis of atypical parkinsonism with corticospinal involvement, a combination suspected to result from a spinocerebellar ataxia or from comorbid parkinsonism and cervical myelopathy. The major pitfall in this case has to do with the interpretation of her slowness, which can be entirely attributable to her severe upper motor neuron syndrome. In pyramidal disorders, slowness is a consequence of impairments in the very source or engine of movements. In this situation, the slowness in alternating movements does not exhibit the *decrement or fatiguing* appreciated in

true parkinsonian bradykinesia, a clinical observation also critical to unraveling Case 19. It is appropriate, then, to add corticospinal dysfunction to the list of causes of pseudo-parkinsonian slowness previously mentioned for cerebellar and dystonic disorders. The "pseudo" prefix is meant to emphasize that, in these disorders, "bradykinesia" is not accompanied by progressive decrement or fatiguing.[1] In addition to her non-decrementing rapid alternating movements of hands and feet, her *purely spastic gait* also exhibited a non-decrementing (i.e., non-festinating) slowness and reduction in stride length, very similar to the *purely rigid gait* of stiff-person syndrome (Video 24b), where fear of falling further contributes to the reduction in gait velocity. Both of these disorders may be mistakenly referred to as parkinsonian.

In the following 2 years, this patient's spasticity and dysarthria worsened substantially. Her speech became unintelligible. L-dopa increases proved of no value. Her brain MRI revealed atrophy of the post-central cortex and the medullary pyramids (Figure 4.3). Injections with botulinum toxin in selected leg muscles allowed preservation of gait with assistance.

These MRI findings[24;25] and her pure upper motor neuron syndrome expressed as progressive spastic quadriparesis and spastic dysarthria met criteria for the clinical diagnosis of primary lateral sclerosis (PLS), a form of motor neuron disease with better prognosis than typical amyotrophic lateral sclerosis.

Discussion: Besides bradykinesia (restriction in the speed of movement) and hypokinesia (restriction in the amplitude of movement), parkinsonian disorders require the ascertainment of progressive *fatiguing or decrement* in repetitive alternating movements during finger or foot tapping. The success in probing this phenomenon depends on asking the patient to make as large and as fast repetitive alternating movements as possible in order to document whether a progressive reduction in amplitude or speed of the movements exists. Some experts believe it is necessary to

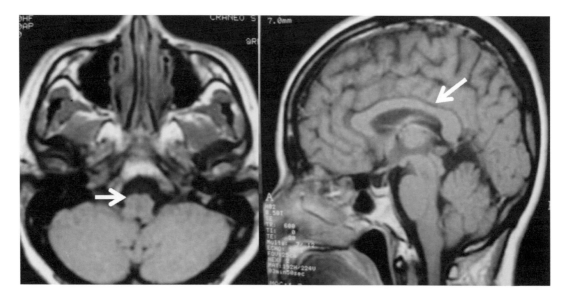

Figure 4.3. T1-weighted axial (left) and mid-sagittal (right) brain MRI demonstrates thinning of the pyramids at the medulla oblongata (horizontal arrow) and at the posterior cross-section in the midbody of the corpus callosum, in the region containing fibers from the paracentral cortical region where the greatest atrophy in primary lateral sclerosis occurs.

observe the patient perform up to 64 repetitions in each limb before this judgment can be made.[1] Most fatiguing, however, manifests early in the tapping task. Furthermore, our own unblinded n-of-2 study, carried out without the confounding of wine intake as we wrote these lines, suggested that the stringent application of this recommendation would yield a high rate of false positive results.

The slowness of movement without fatiguing or decrement is the reason why patients with cerebellar dysfunction, dystonia, and motor neuron disorders may be misdiagnosed as having parkinsonism.[26;27] Disorders that may also be mistakenly labeled as parkinsonism include depression, hypothyroidism, dystonic tremor, frozen shoulder, and catatonia.

Diagnosis: Primary lateral sclerosis

Tip: *The bradykinesia of parkinsonian disorders differs from that of dystonia, cerebellar dysfunction, and pyramidal weakness. A progressive decrement and fatiguing of rapid alternating movements is only appreciated in true parkinsonisms.*

REFERENCES

1. Abdo WF, van de Warrenburg BP, Burn DJ, et al. The clinical approach to movement disorders. *Nat Rev Neurol* 2010;**6**(1):29–37.
2. Albanese A, Lalli S. Is this dystonia? *Mov Disord* 2009;**24**(12):1725–1731.
3. Schwingenschuh P, Ruge D, Edwards MJ, et al. Distinguishing SWEDDs patients with asymmetric resting tremor from Parkinson's disease: a clinical and electrophysiological study. *Mov Disord* 2010;**25**(5):560–569.
4. Schneider SA, Edwards MJ, Mir P, et al. Patients with adult-onset dystonic tremor resembling parkinsonian tremor have scans without evidence of dopaminergic deficit (SWEDDs). *Mov Disord* 2007;**22**(15):2210–2215.
5. Hu WT, Rippon GW, Boeve BF, et al. Alzheimer's disease and corticobasal degeneration presenting as corticobasal syndrome. *Mov Disord* 2009;**24**(9):1375–1379.
6. Ling H, O'Sullivan SS, Holton JL, et al. Does corticobasal degeneration exist? A clinicopathological re-evaluation. *Brain* 2010;**133**(Pt 7):2045–2057.

7. Whitwell JL, Jack CR, Jr., Boeve BF, et al. Imaging correlates of pathology in corticobasal syndrome. *Neurology* 2010;**75**(21):1879–1887.

8. Rohrer JD, Rossor MN, Warren JD. Apraxia in progressive nonfluent aphasia. *J Neurol* 2010;**257**(4): 569–574.

9. Alladi S, Xuereb J, Bak T, et al. Focal cortical presentations of Alzheimer's disease. *Brain* 2007;**130**(Pt 10):2636–2645.

10. Shelley BP, Hodges JR, Kipps CM, et al. Is the pathology of corticobasal syndrome predictable in life? *Mov Disord* 2009;**24**(11):1593–1599.

11. Brennan KC, Jurewicz EC, Ford B, et al. Is essential tremor predominantly a kinetic or a postural tremor? A clinical and electrophysiological study. *Mov Disord* 2002;**17**(2):313–316.

12. Heroux ME, Pari G, Norman KE. The effect of inertial loading on wrist postural tremor in essential tremor. *Clin Neurophysiol* 2009;**120**(5):1020–1029.

13. Arbaizar B, Gomez-Acebo I, Llorca J. Postural induced-tremor in psychiatry. *Psychiatry Clin Neurosci* 2008; **62**(6):638–645.

14. Koller W, Orebaugh C, Lawson L, et al. Pindolol-induced tremor. *Clin Neuropharmacol* 1987; **10**(5):449–452.

15. Morgan JC, Sethi KD. Drug-induced tremors. *Lancet Neurol* 2005;**4**(12):866–876.

16. Maddison P. Neuromyotonia. *Clin Neurophysiol* 2006;**117**(10):2118–2127.

17. Zhang YQ. Teaching video NeuroImages: regional myokymia. *Neurology* 2010;**74**(23):e103–e104.

18. Rueff L, Graber JJ, Bernbaum M, et al. Voltage-gated potassium channel antibody-mediated syndromes: a spectrum of clinical manifestations. *Rev Neurol Dis* 2008;**5**(2):65–72.

19. Vernino S, Auger RG, Emslie-Smith AM, et al. Myasthenia, thymoma, presynaptic antibodies, and a continuum of neuromuscular hyperexcitability. *Neurology* 1999;**53**(6):1233–1239.

20. Matthews PM, Tampieri D, Berkovic SF, et al. Magnetic resonance imaging shows specific abnormalities in the MELAS syndrome. *Neurology* 1991;**41** (7):1043–1046.

21. Zhang XL, Zhang Y, Qiu SJ. Magnetic resonance imaging findings in comparison with histopathology of heroin-associated encephalopathy. *Nan Fang Yi Ke Da Xue Xue Bao* 2007;**27**(2):121–125.

22. Wells EM, Dalmau J. Paraneoplastic neurologic disorders in children. *Curr Neurol Neurosci Rep* 2010; **11**(2):187–194.

23. Kriegstein AR, Shungu DC, Millar WS, et al. Leukoencephalopathy and raised brain lactate from heroin vapor inhalation ("chasing the dragon"). *Neurology* 1999;**53**(8):1765–1773.

24. Smith CD. Serial MRI findings in a case of primary lateral sclerosis. *Neurology* 2002;**58**(4):647–649.

25. Tartaglia MC, Laluz V, Rowe A, et al. Brain atrophy in primary lateral sclerosis. *Neurology* 2009;**72**(14): 1236–1241.

26. Norlinah IM, Bhatia KP, Ostergaard K, et al. Primary lateral sclerosis mimicking atypical parkinsonism. *Mov Disord* 2007;**22**(14):2057–2062.

27. Mabuchi N, Watanabe H, Atsuta N, et al. Primary lateral sclerosis presenting parkinsonian symptoms without nigrostriatal involvement. *J Neurol Neurosurg Psychiatry* 2004;**75**(12):1768–1771.

5

Over-reliance on negative test results

Case 25: Normal cognitive screen in PD

Case: This 64-year-old man developed micrographia, hypophonia, and decreased arm swinging 8 years prior to this evaluation. Treatment with L-dopa restored handwriting and corrected his gait early on. Nevertheless, postural impairment with falls developed 6 years after symptom onset, followed by motor complications in the form of "off" freezing and L-dopa-induced peak-dose dyskinesias, affecting his trunk, arms, and face. Amantadine minimized the peak-dose dyskinesias but a dose above 200 mg/day reliably induced visual hallucinations. Trials with rasagiline first, and ropinirole later, to attenuate the wearing off caused hallucinations and were discontinued. More recently, he had been forgetting names. On two occasions, he could not drive his way to a familiar location without requesting help. He was told to take notes to remember where he parked his car during errands because he has had difficulty finding it in public garages. He and his family were concerned about the possibility of dementia. An office screen showed a Folstein Mini-Mental State Examination (MMSE) score of 27/30. Though corrected with cueing, he could not remember two words at 5 minutes, and made substantial errors in copying the intersecting pentagons (Figure 5.1).

Should we be reassured by his normal MMSE?

The rapid development of hallucinations to different drugs suggested cognitive vulnerability. Perhaps of greater importance was the recent difficulty in

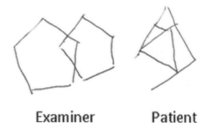

Examiner   **Patient**

Figure 5.1. Performance of the intersecting pentagon figure-copying task.

orienting himself in relatively familiar environments. This impairment of visuospatial orientation is an important historical piece in, and can predate, PD dementia (PDD).[1] Despite a score within the normal range for MMSE, the abnormal intercepting pentagons task unveiled this problem. Finally, this man has the postural instability-gait disorder (PIGD) variant of PD, which is known to pose a greater risk of developing into PDD than the tremor-dominant type.[2]

How best to properly assess the cognitive function and the risk of dementia?

In this setting, a proper screen should include the administration of the Montreal Cognitive Assessment (MoCA). The MoCA probes visuospatial and constructional praxis as well as word list generation, important elements of the cognitive vulnerability of PD. A re-evaluation 6 months later disclosed a stable MMSE at 27/30 but a MoCA score of 23/30. He made mistakes in the Trail-Making Test part of the MoCA and the cube, in the serial sevens, and fell short of the 11 F-words requested.

For both MMSE and MoCA, cognitive impairment is generally defined as a score < 26. He was therefore considered normal per MMSE, but cognitively impaired per MoCA. The diagnosis of multiple-domain mild cognitive impairment (PD-MCI) was made. Three years later, there was documentation of impairment in social functioning that met the final criterion for the diagnosis of PDD.

Discussion: Two clinical pearls and one major pitfall in the diagnosis of MCI and PDD are worth emphasizing in relationship with this case. First, many more PD patients exist with deficits in executive function than with dementia, implying that executive dysfunction alone is not a sensitive marker of dementia risk. This is presumably the result of near universal impairment of dopaminergic, frontostriatal circuits. It follows that the state of dopaminergic treatment affects the performance of frontally-mediated, executive function-probing tasks such as working memory, planning, and attentional set shifting. Second, fewer patients have visuospatial and verbal fluency impairments but these deficits are disproportionately common among those who go on to develop dementia. PD patients at risk for dementia are most impaired on tests of semantic fluency and visuospatial and constructional dysfunction, which localize to posterior cortical rather than frontostriatal networks.[3] The major pitfall is that the widely used MMSE does little to distinguish either of the two groups and, thus, is expected to be rather insensitive to timely identification of those with mild cognitive impairment marching onto dementia. Approximately half of PD patients with a normal MMSE score (>26) have impaired cognitive impairment based on a similar MoCA cutoff score.[4;5] Therefore MoCA is more sensitive than MMSE and provides a more reliable assessment of the risk of dementia in PD. This patient's PIGD motor phenotype and his poor word fluency and pentagon copying skills defined a motor-and-cognitive profile at increased risk of

subsequently developing dementia, which was eventually confirmed.[3;6] The MoCA falls short in not probing the semantic fluency, integrated in the left medial temporal lobe, whose impairment appears to be more predictive of cognitive decline and dementia in PD than its phonemic counterpart, which is more diffusely integrated in the frontal and temporal lobes.

Diagnosis: PD-MCI preceding PDD

Tip: *Inability to copy intersecting pentagons and reduced (semantic) word list generation are important early cognitive impairments among those at high risk of developing PDD. The MMSE is rather insensitive in identifying this subgroup.*

Case 26: Comatose movements and undetermined pleocytosis

Case: This previously healthy 26-year-old African-American woman presented to the emergency department after an acute episode of psychotic behavior while at work where she was described as becoming abruptly "agitated and restless." Over the next few days, she developed seizures and impairment of consciousness for which she required intubation and intensive care monitoring. She showed intermittent agitation with screaming and crying spells. EEG revealed bilateral independent temporal epileptiform discharges which prompted treatment with phenytoin. On neurological examination, she was awake but unresponsive to verbal or noxious stimulation. She had choreiform movements of the face and disorganized but conjugate eye movements (Video 26). A brain MRI was negative but CSF examination showed lymphocytic pleocytosis. An extensive search for viral etiologies was negative. She did not respond to treatment with acyclovir.

Is this just a case of aseptic meningoencephalitis?

Lymphocytic pleocytosis does not imply that the encephalitis is necessarily viral nor that it has to be "aseptic." When Movement Disorders neurologists get summoned to an ICU bed, the commonest reasons are generalized rigidity with tremor (probably neuroleptic malignant syndrome), leg-predominant rigidity with myoclonus (possibly serotonin syndrome), or some form of oromandibular dystonia (likely an acute dystonic reaction). None of these entail lymphocytic pleocytosis. Herpes simplex virus, responsible for 10% of endemic cases of viral encephalitis in the US, rarely presents with any movement disorder. Only Japanese B encephalitis, the most common epidemic encephalitis outside North America, is known to cause abnormal movements, typically parkinsonism and dystonia given its tropism to the substantia nigra and basal ganglia.[7]

What are key descriptors that reveal the underlying pathology?

The key elements in the history are "wakeful unresponsiveness," abnormal movements, and psychotic/epileptic outbreaks. An encephalopathic process associated with any movement disorder in the context of "wakeful unresponsiveness" should raise the consideration of ovarian teratomas often due to anti-NMDA-receptor (NMDAR) antibodies.[8] This etiology may well be more common than herpes simplex virus given our local registry and the vast experience accumulated by Dalmau and colleagues within a few years.[9]

This patient had a negative abdominal ultrasound and pelvis CT. Strong suspicion for anti-NMDA-receptor encephalitis prompted a pelvic MRI which demonstrated a right ovarian mass only on fat suppression sequences, which proved to be a teratoma. Surgical excision of this teratoma and intravenous methylprednisolone led to noticeable improvement in function over the next few days. Five weeks after this treatment, the patient returned to work.

Discussion: Ovarian teratoma-associated anti-NMDAR encephalitis has become the most common intersection between the roads of epilepsy, psychiatry, and movement disorders. Abnormal movements tend to more commonly affect the trunk and face, particularly in the form of jaw dystonia and bucco-lingual-facial dyskinesias, paroxysmal opisthotonus, catatonic postures, and unusual stereotypic limb movements.[10] Young African-American women are a particularly vulnerable demographic. Teratomas tend to be discovered more frequently among those 18 years or older. Patients treated with tumor resection and immunotherapy (corticosteroids, intravenous immunoglobulin, or plasma exchange) respond faster to treatment and less frequently need second-line immunotherapy (cyclophosphamide or rituximab, or both) than do patients without a tumor who receive similar initial immunotherapy.[9] It is sobering to appreciate that over one fourth of all unexplained new-onset epileptic encephalopathies in young women, especially when heralded by psychiatric symptoms, are due to NMDAR antibodies.[11] Hypofunctioning of the NMDAR is likely to underlie the psychosis of patients with anti-NMDAR encephalitis since NMDAR agonists ameliorate psychotic symptoms.

Diagnosis: Anti-NMDAR encephalitis

Tip: *NMDA receptor encephalitis is a treatable autoimmune, sometimes paraneoplastic disorder, likely under-recognized as "aseptic meningoencephalitis." Psychosis and seizures leading to a state of unresponsive wakefulness, in the presence of any movement disorder, are important clinical clues.*

Case 27: Feeding dystonia with a negative diagnostic test

Contributed by Dr. Ruth Walker, Bronx, New York

Case: This 31-year-old man reported abnormalities of his gait and involuntary movements, especially when nervous, for the past 3 years. There was a distant cousin on the paternal side of the family with a similar disorder, although further details were not known. He had a 26-year-old brother who was in good health. There was no consanguinity. At the age of 20, he developed depression and visual hallucinations, and was diagnosed variously with schizophrenia and bipolar disease. He also had frequent vocal tics, and his head pulled to the

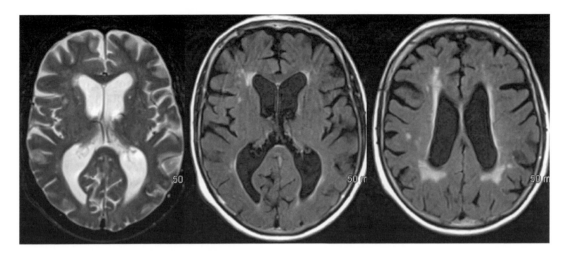

Figure 5.2. Axial T2-weighted (left) and FLAIR (center and right) brain MRI showing moderate cortical atrophy as well as mild caudate atrophy. Patchy periventricular white matter disease can be appreciated.

right, especially when eating. Eating was complicated by spitting and drooling. He bit his tongue and the inside of his mouth. He had lost weight and was occasionally falling. He had become clumsy and frequently dropped things. He was forgetful and showed poor judgment, such as when crossing the street. He has some obsessive behaviors, including compulsive shopping. He tended to be depressed, lonely, and distrustful of other people. He had never had seizures.

Does his examination confirm "feeding dystonia"?

Although his chorea and dystonia were generalized, there was predominant involvement of the orolingual-buccal region (Video 27a). He exhibited mild tongue thrusting when chewing. Speech was mildly dysarthric. Reflexes were absent throughout and plantar responses were flexor. Vibration sense was mildly decreased at both ankles. He had difficulty maintaining posture for even a few seconds. Gait was bizarre and poorly coordinated with dystonic posturing of both feet and frequent leg buckling.

This clinical picture is strongly suggestive of chorea-acanthocytosis.

What other supportive finding do we need?

In chorea-acanthocytosis, the brain MRI is a critical piece of information (Figure 5.2). It demonstrated generalized atrophy with ex-vacuo hydrocephalus and mild atrophy in the caudate nucleus. In this setting, Huntington's disease is also an important consideration. Indeed, genetic testing ruled out HD and additional investigations excluded antiphospholipid antibody syndrome, hypoparathyroidism, hypercalcemia, and Wilson's disease. However, one could strongly argue that these tests were unnecessary and might have been delayed until chorea-acanthocytosis was adequately excluded given the classical clinical picture. To clinch the diagnosis of chorea-acanthocytosis, creatine kinase and a blood smear to look for acanthocytes were requested. CK was elevated (1240 IU/L) but acanthocytes were not identified.

Lacking acanthocytes, should the diagnostic effort move elsewhere?

Chorea with an orolingual-buccal dystonia component is typically secondary or heredodegenerative, almost never a primary form of dystonia. Given a relatively short differential in the setting of caudate atrophy, hyperCKemia, and negative Huntington's disease genetic testing, chorea-acanthocytosis should be pursued further – even in the setting of no acanthocytes in peripheral blood.

Chorein Western blot (Munich, Germany) demonstrated low expression of chorein supporting the clinical diagnosis of chorea-acanthocytosis (ChAc).

Discussion: The differential diagnosis for chorea and dystonia with a predominant orolingual-buccal component is short. It includes ChAc, pantothenate kinase-associated neurodegeneration, neuroferritinopathy, Wilson's disease, Lesch-Nyhan syndrome, acquired hepatolenticular degeneration, and postanoxic and tardive dyskinesia.[12] Additional clinical or imaging features help in diagnosing each of these. Tardive dystonia and dyskinesia due to chronic exposure to neuroleptics can mimic ChAc. However, in tardive dyskinesia as in most of the disorders listed above, tongue involvement manifests as spontaneous protrusion (Video 27b). It is only in ChAc where the tongue dystonia is task-specific, most obvious when placing solid food into the mouth, and with chewing and swallowing food. As such, this action-induced feeding dystonia has been considered highly specific for ChAc.[13] In this situation, despite the absence of acanthocytes, it was appropriate to pursue sequencing of the *VPS13A* gene or examine for the absence of its protein product, chorein, on Western blot.[14] An important diagnostic pitfall is to assume that acanthocytes will be universally present in a disease honoring its name. Not only can acanthocytes be absent or appear very late in the course of the disease but their identification is notoriously unreliable by standard laboratory procedures. To enhance the detection of acanthocytes it is recommended to dilute blood 1:1 with 0.9% saline and 10 U/mL heparin. Review using phase-contrast microscopy is undertaken after the sample has been incubated in a shaker for 30 minutes.[15] Another pitfall is the absence of seizures by history. Adding seizures to his chorea with orolingual-buccal predominance would have made the diagnosis all but certain from the outset. Regardless, the bulk of the evidence pointed in the direction of ChAc and a definitive diagnostic test was begging to be carried out despite the negative screening tests.

Diagnosis: Chorea-acanthocytosis

Tip: *The absence of acanthocytes, especially on first screen, should not detract from pursuing the diagnosis of ChAc in appropriate clinical circumstances.*

Case 28: B₁₂-deficiency ataxia with normal B₁₂ levels?

Case: This 37-year-old woman with a previous history of hypothyroidism and depression developed numbness and tingling that extended from the fingertips to the upper arms about 4 months prior to this evaluation. Subsequently, these symptoms extended into her legs. She could no longer run a mile and was losing her balance. On exam, there was mild dysmetria on heel-to-shin and impairment in tandem gait, with a slight delay in the relaxation phase of the muscle stretch reflexes and reduced vibratory and position sense in her feet. Romberg sign was present. Evaluation showed a normal brain and spine MRI. There was mild anemia. Metabolic screen with fasting glucose, thyroid panel, renal and liver functions, as well as B_{12} and vitamin E were negative. Her hypothyroidism was adequately controlled.

What is the predominant deficit? Why is the screening insufficient?

The main problem is a sensory ataxia due to posterior column dysfunction, manifested by proprioceptive and vibratory loss and a positive Romberg sign. In this situation, and because of the high probability of a metabolic disorder, vitamin B_{12} level is insufficient to screen for its deficiency, particularly in the face of anemia.

Do we just retest vitamin B₁₂ levels?

In subtle deficiency, B_{12} levels may remain in the low–normal range of 200 to 300 pg/mL (150 to 220 pmol/L). Also associated liver disease can lead

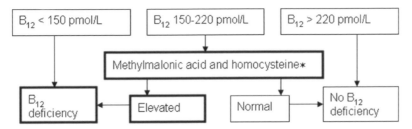

Figure 5.3. Serum homocysteine and methylmalonic acid levels can help define true deficiency and replace the Schilling test and the antibodies against parietal cells (non-specific) and against intrinsic factor (insensitive) in the diagnosis of B_{12} deficiency. In severe cases ($B_{12} < 100$ pmol/L) there may also be macrocytic anemia with hypersegmentation of neutrophils, pancytopenia, and signs of ineffective erythropoiesis (high lactate dehydrogenase and indirect bilirubin).[16]

to falsely low–normal or normal levels of vitamin B_{12}. To uncover true vitamin B_{12} deficiency (and distinguish it from folate deficiency), homocysteine and methylmalonic acid levels should be measured (Figure 5.3). In vitamin B_{12} deficiency, the levels of both homocysteine and methylmalonic acid are elevated, whereas in most cases of folate deficiency only the homocysteine level is increased. Methylmalonic acid concentration reflects intracellular vitamin B_{12} stores and exhibits higher specificity for low vitamin B_{12} status than any other metabolite including homocysteine.

Both methylmalonic acid and homocysteine were increased, confirming vitamin B_{12} deficiency. Since this patient reported eating meat and dairy products, malabsorption of vitamin B_{12} was deemed more likely than poor intake. In the absence of a history of gastrointestinal surgery or drugs that inhibit gastric acid secretion, the most likely cause of this patient's inability to absorb vitamin B_{12} is pernicious anemia. The patient received 1 mg of parenteral vitamin B_{12} daily for 1 week, followed by weekly injections for 2 months, and 1 mg orally per day thereafter. She had complete recovery of her deficits.

Discussion: Vitamin B_{12} (cobalamin) deficiency may present with symmetric paresthesias and signs of sensory ataxia due to proprioceptive impairment affecting the lower, and to a lesser extent, upper limbs. This diagnosis can be reached in the setting of normal B_{12} levels and even in the absence of overt anemia. The true underlying disorder was only revealed after

confirming elevated levels of methylmalonic acid and homocysteine. This patient was at increased risk for this disorder given her history of hypothyroidism. Both hypothyroidism and vitamin B_{12} deficiency may indicate a more widespread autoimmune disorder (such as autoimmune polyendocrine syndrome type IIIB, which consists of autoimmune thyroiditis and pernicious anemia, as may be the case in this patient). In addition to proprioceptive loss, important clues for ataxias due to sensory neuropathies include hypo- or arreflexia, painful dysesthesias, worsening coordination on eye closure, and pseudoathetosis. Imaging may demonstrate T2-weighted hyperintensity in the posterior columns of the spinal cord with or without some atrophy. Electrophysiological studies may show diffuse absence or severely decreased amplitude of sensory nerve action potentials and undetectable or abnormal somatosensory evoked potentials.[17]

The differential diagnosis of sensory ataxias requires separating posterior column myelopathies, sensory ganglionopathies (non-length-dependent proprioceptive and vibratory sensory deprivation),[18] and demyelinating autoimmune polyneuropathies (Table 5.1). Sensory ataxias are not an early manifestation of axonal distal peripheral neuropathies.

Diagnosis: Sensory ataxia due to vitamin B_{12} deficiency

Tip: *Increased methylmalonic acid and homocysteine may be the only abnormalities associated*

Table 5.1. (Non-cerebellar) sensory ataxias

Localization	Classification	Etiologies
Posterior column	Myelopathies	**Friedreich ataxia** **Metabolic** (vitamin B_{12} deficiency,* folate deficiency,* vitamin E deficiency,* copper deficiency,* POLG1 mutation) **Toxic** (nitrous oxide myeloneuropathy,* Clioquinol [antiprotozoal hydroxyquinoline], cassava ingestion) **Infectious** (HIV and HTLV myelopathies, tabes dorsalis) Compressive/vascular myelopathy
Sensory ganglia	Sensory neuronopathies or ganglionopathies	**Metabolic** (thiamine [B_1] deficiency**) **Paraneoplastic** (Subacute sensory neuronopathy due to anti-Hu and anti-CV2/CRMP5 antibodies) **Autoimmune** (Sjögren's syndrome, Miller Fisher syndrome; and Bickerstaff's brainstem encephalitis) **Drugs** (cisplatin, pyridoxine [B_6] intoxication) **Inherited** disorders with degeneration of dorsal root ganglion cells.
Peripheral nerves	Immune-mediated *demyelinating* neuropathies-polyradiculopathies	Ataxic variant of Guillain-Barré syndrome: Miller Fisher syndrome (Anti-GQ1b), sensory ataxic neuropathy (Anti-GD1b), anti-MAG neuropathy

* Vitamin B_{12}, vitamin E, folate, and copper deficiencies as well as nitrous oxide intoxication may present with a picture reflecting myeloneuropathy or subacute combined degeneration of the spinal cord (pyramidal, cerebellar, and neuropathic signs). Folate supplementation alone improves the anemia and peripheral neuropathy of B_{12} deficiency but not any CNS manifestations. Vitamin E deficiency is similar to Friedreich ataxia plus retinopathy.
** CNS manifestations of thiamine deficiency include Wernicke encephalopathy (Case 1) and optic neuropathy. Other manifestations include axonal peripheral neuropathy (*dry beriberi*), in severe cases mimicking the axonal type of Guillain-Barré syndrome, and high-output heart failure (wet beriberi). MAG: myelin-associated-glycoprotein.

with sensory ataxia due to vitamin B_{12} deficiency. Proprioceptive loss and Romberg sign exculpate the cerebellum from wrongdoing as the cause of the ataxia.

REFERENCES

1. Huber SJ, Shuttleworth EC, Freidenberg DL. Neuro-psychological differences between the dementias of Alzheimer's and Parkinson's diseases. *Arch Neurol* 1989;**46**(12):1287–1291.
2. Alves G, Wentzel-Larsen T, Aarsland D, et al. Progression of motor impairment and disability in Parkinson disease: a population-based study. *Neurology* 2005;**65** (9):1436–1441.
3. Williams-Gray CH, Foltynie T, Brayne CE, et al. Evolution of cognitive dysfunction in an incident Parkinson's disease cohort. *Brain* 2007;**130**(Pt 7): 1787–1798.
4. Zadikoff C, Fox SH, Tang-Wai DF, et al. A comparison of the mini mental state exam to the Montreal cognitive assessment in identifying cognitive deficits in Parkinson's disease. *Mov Disord* 2008;**23**(2):297–299.
5. Nazem S, Siderowf AD, Duda JE, et al. Montreal cognitive assessment performance in patients with Parkinson's disease with "normal" global cognition according to mini-mental state examination score. *J Am Geriatr Soc* 2009;**57**(2):304–308.
6. Williams-Gray CH, Evans JR, Goris A, et al. The distinct cognitive syndromes of Parkinson's disease: 5 year follow-up of the CamPaIGN cohort. *Brain* 2009;**132** (Pt 11):2958–2969.

7. Misra UK, Kalita J. Spectrum of movement disorders in encephalitis. *J Neurol* 2010;**257**(12):2052–2058.

8. Kleinig TJ, Thompson PD, Matar W, et al. The distinctive movement disorder of ovarian teratoma-associated encephalitis. *Mov Disord* 2008;**23**(9):1256–1261.

9. Dalmau J, Lancaster E, Martinez-Hernandez E, et al. Clinical experience and laboratory investigations in patients with anti-NMDAR encephalitis. *Lancet Neurol* 2011;**10**(1):63–74.

10. Ferioli S, Dalmau J, Kobet CA, et al. Anti-N-methyl-D-aspartate receptor encephalitis: characteristic behavioral and movement disorder. *Arch Neurol* 2010;**67**(2):250–251.

11. Niehusmann P, Dalmau J, Rudlowski C, et al. Diagnostic value of N-methyl-D-aspartate receptor antibodies in women with new-onset epilepsy. *Arch Neurol* 2009;**66**(4):458–464.

12. Schneider SA, Aggarwal A, Bhatt M, et al. Severe tongue protrusion dystonia: clinical syndromes and possible treatment. *Neurology* 2006;**67**(6):940–943.

13. Bader B, Walker RH, Vogel M, et al. Tongue protrusion and feeding dystonia: a hallmark of chorea-acanthocytosis. *Mov Disord* 2010;**25**(1):127–129.

14. Dobson-Stone C, Velayos-Baeza A, Filippone LA, et al. Chorein detection for the diagnosis of chorea-acanthocytosis. *Ann Neurol* 2004;**56**(2):299–302.

15. Dobson-Stone C, Rampoldi L, Bader B, et al. Chorea-acanthocytosis. In: Pagon RA, Bird TD, Dolan CR, Stephens K, eds. *SourceGeneReviews* [Internet]. Seattle (WA): University of Washington, Seattle; 1993-2002, Jun 14 [updated 2011 Aug 18].

16. Marks PW, Zukerberg LR. Case records of the Massachusetts General Hospital. Weekly clinicopathological exercises. Case 30–2004. A 37-year-old woman with paresthesias of the arms and legs. *N Engl J Med* 2004;**351**(13):1333–1341.

17. Spinazzi M, Angelini C, Patrini C. Subacute sensory ataxia and optic neuropathy with thiamine deficiency. *Nat Rev Neurol* 2010;**6**(5):288–293.

18. Kuntzer T, Antoine JC, Steck AJ. Clinical features and pathophysiological basis of sensory neuronopathies (ganglionopathies). *Muscle Nerve* 2004;**30**(3):255–268.

6

Failure of pattern recognition

Unlike prior chapters, this section concentrates on pattern recognition of abnormal movements as the method for providing the highest diagnostic yield – if appropriately interpreted. Pattern recognition may be dismissed as a gut-over-mind strategy, and one that can lead to diagnostic errors, as will be shown in the following cases. However, patients affected with movement disorders will inevitably trigger memories of "that particular case," where a *pattern* was generated that would explain all similarly looking presentations in the future. Because some of these pitfalls are among the most common diagnostic carcasses in the graveyard of a neurologist's misdiagnoses, attention to detail is paramount.

For the following cases, the reader will be directed to the video cases first – with elements of the history, relatively secondary for the diagnosis, provided later only to confirm or correct the reader's heuristic assessment.

Case 29: Facial and neck dystonia in PD

Case: This 49-year-old man developed PD symptoms, starting with right-hand resting tremor, 18 years prior to this evaluation. He was referred for consideration of botulinum toxin injections in selected facial muscles (Video 29a).

What pattern may have been missed?

There was *painful* oromandibular dystonia and blepharospasm, present at rest but worse during action

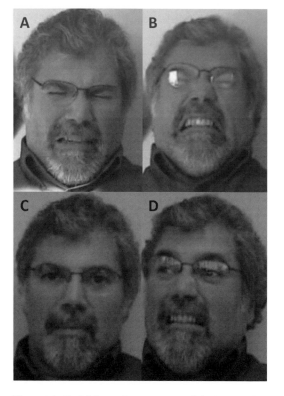

Figure 6.1. Facial dystonia at rest (A) and during speech (B) before and after (C and D, respectively) reduction of DBS stimulation rate.

(Figure 6.1, A–B). Speech was dysarthric and had a spastic component. Both arms showed dystonia when held outstretched. This pattern of focal dystonia is unlike that of most primary and secondary dystonias – particularly because of the associated pain (unusual in focal or segmental dystonias outside the cervical region) and the excessive effort to speak and open the eyes. Had we not known that this patient had PD we could not have made the connection in the absence of parkinsonian signs.

Could this phenotype be a complication of treatment?

Indeed. He underwent subthalamic deep brain stimulation (STN DBS) implantation 8 years previously, with substantial benefit. His stimulators were turned off once or twice in the past and his tremor and rigidity clearly worsened. His stimulation parameters were believed to be optimized. However, his speech had gradually deteriorated over the years. Although his wife indicated that facial pain and "contortions" were of concern for at least 2 years, no connection was made with the surgical treatment. In fact, the problem was categorized as a dose-limiting side effect of his medication regimen.

His current was reduced by half by lowering the rate from 185 to 90 Hz while keeping the amplitude (3.5 V) and pulse width (60 μs) the same. His blepharospasm and pain disappeared and the resting component of his oromandibular dystonia markedly abated (Video 29b) (Figure 6.1, C–D). Further improvements took place in subsequent weeks.

Discussion: Painful facial dystonia and spastic dysarthria are relatively uncommon but recognized complications of STN DBS.[1] It must be noted that although these complications are often ascertained at the time of dose titration, they may present many years later, once the stimulator settings are deemed "optimized," as in this case. The long latency from STN DBS implantation to the development of this motor complication translated into a low index of suspicion for the dystonia to represent a side effect of stimulation. Incorrect assumptions about its nature led inevitably to a delay in the appropriate corrective action. This stimulation-induced dystonia only requires downward adjustments in amplitude or rate. There is no need to proceed with

botulinum toxin injections unless adjustments in stimulator settings were to become impossible due to intolerable loss of motor benefits. A distinct, relatively fixed dystonia involving the oromandibular region has been reported in PD as a severe "off" manifestation, responding nicely to subcutaneous apomorphine.[2] This is in contrast with the more choreic involvement of this region and neck seen as L-dopa-induced peak-dose dyskinesia. Finally, in someone with a much shorter disease duration than this patient, without having undergone STN DBS implantation, one needs to distinguish this form of "off" facial dystonia from that due to L-dopa in MSA patients,[3;4] which is typically painless and may respond to sensory tricks (Case 13c).

Diagnosis: Stimulation-induced facial dystonia in a patient with PD

Tip: *STN DBS can induce late complications, including focal dystonia and spasticity, which can be corrected with adjustment of stimulator settings.*

Case 30: When familial alcohol-responsive tremor is not ET

Case: This 69-year-old woman first noted very mild hand tremor as far back as 50 years ago. She had very little in the way of difficulties until about 2 years ago, when she noticed that the tremor had worsened. Her handwriting became a casualty with extreme difficulty to write. Moving the mouse and typing was difficult due to jitteriness, though she did not feel inaccuracy. She had also begun to spill fluid from cups and was avoiding using a spoon for soup. She resorted to using a straw for drinking most fluids. She had noted no head tremor and was unaware of any voice tremor. She felt the tremor affected both hands about equally and did not involve her legs or feet. The tremor was exclusively present during action; never at rest. She was on both primidone and propranolol at high doses without side effects or benefits. She had several family members with similar tremor (father, older sister, brother). Alcohol improved her tremor but she kept sober after treatment for alcoholism.

Table 6.1. Clinical features more common in essential tremor (ET) and dystonic tremor (DyT)

More common in ET	Do not help distinguish ET from DyT	More common in DyT
Younger age at onset	Response to alcohol	Older age at onset
Combined head, arms, and voice tremor	Family history	*Isolated* head tremor
	Isolated voice tremor*	

Adapted from Schrag et al.[5] and Jain et al.[6]

* Voice tremor was non-significantly more common among "atypical" tremor (e.g., dystonia) in the Schrag et al. series.

What does the story suggest? Was the examination supportive of the presumptive diagnosis?

This long-standing, alcohol-responsive, familial tremor appears to be nothing but ET. Indeed the examination showed a relatively rhythmic postural and kinetic tremor of the hands, with a tremor component also in her voice. Of interest, the tremor increased with resistance, as shown when testing her strength (Video 30a). Her gait showed normal arm swing without tremor but some impairment of tandem and postural reflexes. All these features were interpreted as being supportive of the diagnostic impression generated with the history.

Will the treatment response and evolution also be supportive?

Propranolol was titrated to 360 mg/day but discontinued for lack of efficacy. Primidone, introduced later, was titrated to 750 mg/day to no avail and was discontinued. A trial with clonazepam yielded no benefits. Two years later, her tremor had worsened further in the hands and, more noticeable later, in the head. On re-examination, she had a jerky head tremor and increased amplitude of the asymmetric hand tremor, which had become jerkier. Of interest, the patient demonstrated that changes in position of the arm altered the magnitude of the tremor (Video 30b). These changes helped revise the diagnostic impression from ET to dystonic tremor. A combination of trihexyphenidyl and clonazepam brought the tremor under better control.

Discussion: Essential tremor is definitely an overused label. Anywhere from 40 to 50% of those diagnosed with ET may actually have other conditions, most often PD or, as in this case, dystonia.[5;6] Although neither response to alcohol nor family history reliably distinguish ET from dystonic tremor, certain features may be more common in one compared to the other (Table 6.1). Still, some clinical features of ET, PD, and dystonic tremor overlap. For example, ET tremor can present unilaterally and at rest, becoming potentially misdiagnosed as PD (see Case 15), or with jerky handwriting and be misdiagnosed as dystonic tremor (Videos 30c, 30d) (Figure 6.2). Dystonia, as the second most common source of "false ET," tends to produce a tremor that, when in full bloom, should be very different from ET: asymmetric, dysrhythmic, irregular in amplitude and periodicity, directional (i.e., more overt in a given direction), and *exacerbated by muscle contraction.*[7] Dystonia is easier to identify when the tremor appears or increases only on certain positions or tasks, when overt posturing develops (e.g., "spooning" of the hands, that is, wrist flexion with hyperextension of the fingers when arms are outstretched), and in the setting of clear sensory tricks (e.g., touching the more affected hand with the contralateral one to lessen the amplitude of the tremor). *Isolated* tremor in the legs, head, facial muscles, voice, jaw, or tongue is considered atypical for ET and most often indicative of parkinsonism or dystonia.

The observation that the tremor amplitude increased in this patient when performing strength testing at the initial visit (Video 30a) is a potentially useful application of the concept that dystonic tremor is exacerbated by muscle contraction. Indeed, application of resistance, weight, or "inertial loading" is known to reduce postural tremor in

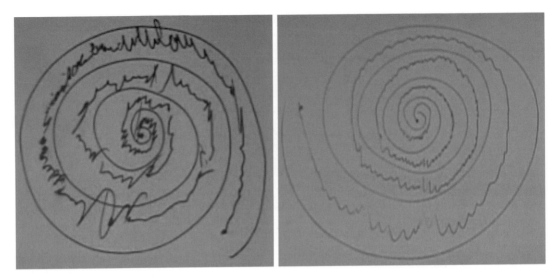

Figure 6.2. Spiral drawing task before (left) and 4 months later (right), after primidone was titrated to a dose of 300 mg/day in a 76-year-old man with ET. The initial jerky pattern is replaced by a more ET-like sinusoidal waveform.

ET and PD but not in dystonic tremor or enhanced physiologic tremor.[8] We have previously reported a patient with "presumed ET" in whom tremor was brought out exclusively by carrying a weight.[9] This patient also had a "no-no" head tremor with mild left torticollis and laterocollis, suggesting that dystonia was the underlying disorder.

Diagnosis: Dystonic tremor

Tip: *Jerky irregular tremor following the "dystonia rules" (directionality, poor rhythmicity, and position- or task-specific) define dystonic tremor. Dystonic tremor is often misdiagnosed as essential tremor, especially in individuals with family history and response to alcohol. Alcohol response can be seen in another disorder often mistaken for ET, myoclonus dystonia.*

Case 31: Rhythmic facial movements

Case: This 41-year-old patient developed diplopia, unsteadiness, and weight loss. Examination showed rhythmic contractions of the face and platysma, associated with abnormal spontaneous eye movements and left blepharospasm (Video 31a). There was

complete supranuclear vertical and, to a lesser extent, horizontal gaze palsy. Note his impaired horizontal pursuit and complete inability to initiate vertical gaze. These deficits were overcome by oculocephalic maneuvers.

What disorders should this movement pattern bring to mind?

Technically this pattern of movements is only characteristic of one disease, Whipple's disease, and no differential exists. The pendular vergence oscillations of the eyes and synchronous contractions of the masticatory but not palatal muscles qualify for the label of oculomasticatory myorhythmia (OMM) (Figure 6.3). This patient became symptom free after 6 months of antibiotic treatment. A presentation without the synchronous ocular movements is also uniquely associated with Whipple's if the supranuclear vertical and horizontal gaze palsy are documented (Video 31b).

Discussion: OMM is pathognomonic of Whipple's disease.[10] In its presence, neither jejunal biopsy nor blood or cerebrospinal fluid polymerase chain

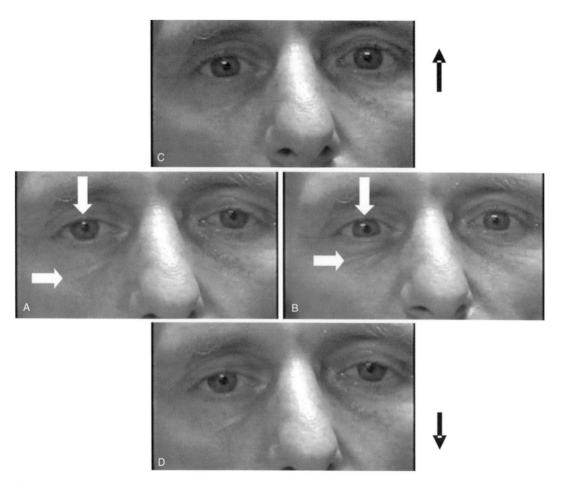

Figure 6.3. Divergent (A) and convergent (B) ocular oscillations can be appreciated in primary gaze (the corneal light is displaced laterally from A to B). Note the elevation of the inferior eyelid crease (horizontal arrow, A to B), synchronous with the convergent ocular movements. Patient shows marked restriction of upgaze (C) and downgaze (D) (Taken with permission from Revilla et al.[14]).

reaction of *Tropheryma whippelii* is necessary for the initiation of trimethoprim-sulfamethoxazole.[11] Myorhythmia applies to slow, 1-to-2 Hz rhythmic, tremor-like contractions of any muscle groups. Without the topographical specificity to the facial region and the concurrent ocular movements, the differential of this disorder does expand beyond Whipple's disease. Non-oculomasticatory myorhythmia most often develops with lesions in the central tegmental tract component of the Guillain-Mollaret triangle, the white matter pathways connecting the inferior olives, dentate nuclei, and red nuclei in each side. The critical structures responsible for the development of this movement, however, are not well understood. In these cases, myorhythmia may involve the palate (in the form of a palatal tremor, formerly referred to as palatal myoclonus) and unilateral arm. Causative lesions include brainstem strokes, demyelination, trauma, chronic nutritional deficiencies, phenytoin intoxication, limbic encephalitis, (*Listeria*) rhombencephalitis, and Hashimoto encephalopathy. The

Table 6.2. Range of motor complications

Primarily "Off" state	Primarily "On" state	Intermediary state
Predictable wearing off	Peak-dose dyskinesias	Diphasic dyskinesias (end- and
Random "off" state	(monophasic dyskinesias)	beginning-of-dose)
"Off" dystonia	"On" freezing (rare)	Rapid on–off fluctuations
Freezing of gait	Myoclonus (from levodopa or amantadine)	Yo-yo-ing
Delayed "on"		Sudden "off" state

Adapted from Fox and Lang, 2008,[19] and Espay, 2010.[18]

involved palate and arm are ipsilateral to the affected dentate nucleus or superior cerebellar peduncle lesions or contralateral to a typically hypertrophic (denervated) inferior olive.[12;13] Cerebellar ataxia is almost always part of the presentation.

Diagnosis: Whipple's disease

Tip: *Oculomasticatory myorhythmia is pathognomonic for Whipple's disease. Only myorhythmia without the "oculo" part and without the supranuclear gaze palsy extends the differential beyond T. whippelii and into the realm of lesions in the central tegmental tract, or, less commonly, dentate nucleus or superior cerebellar peduncle.*

Case 32: Dyskinesias with a "restless leg" pattern

Contributed by Dr. Leo Verhagen, Chicago, Illinois
   Case: This 45-year-old man with 12 years of PD had developed dyskinesias as part of his motor complications (Video 32). He had been decreasing the dose of L-dopa but this approach was not helping.

What is the clue that these were not typical L-dopa-induced dyskinesias?

The first is that he was probably getting worse as the L-dopa dose was being reduced, which would not have been expected for the more common peak-dose variant of this motor complication. The earlier, more important clinical clue to appreciate, which would have averted the

worsening documented with a dose-reduction strategy, was the prominent involvement of the legs, exhibiting ballistic movements conveying a severe "restless leg" appearance (more often, patients do not endorse such a manifestation). This pattern of diphasic dyskinesias often goes underappreciated by clinicians and patients, especially if management decisions are made by phone. Unlike the more common peak-dose, upper-body predominant dyskinesias, the diphasic or end-of-dose variant is treated by raising the dopaminergic stimulation. This particular individual improved dramatically a few minutes after a subcutaneous injection of apomorphine.

Discussion: Monophasic or peak-dose dyskinesias are classically recognized by the appearance of choreic movements of the trunk, arms, and neck, during the period of maximum (supra)therapeutic efficacy of dopaminergic drugs (Figure 6.4, A–B).[15] These movements are present at rest but substantially worsen with action, while speaking, or during stress.[16] Conversely, diphasic or beginning- and end-of-dose dyskinesias manifest as ballistic or stereotypic paddling or kicking movements of the legs, arising at a transitional state between the "off" and "on" states (Figure 6.4C). Within this transitional state, rapid "on–off" fluctuations and "yo-yo-ing" can arise (Table 6.2). The latter applies to the presence of both "off" (e.g., tremor) and "on" phenomena (including monophasic dyskinesias) within a very short time so as to virtually appear concurrently rather than sequentially. The peak-dose and diphasic dyskinesias have a differential

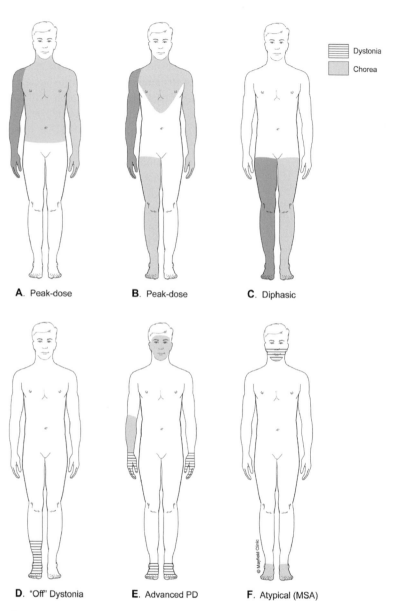

Dystonia

Chorea

A. Peak-dose   **B**. Peak-dose   **C**. Diphasic

D. "Off" Dystonia   **E**. Advanced PD   **F**. Atypical (MSA)

Figure 6.4. Typical topographic patterns among various forms of dyskinesia in PD. Right-sided onset of disease is assumed for all cases. A. Peak-dose levodopa-induced dyskinesias tend to involve the upper trunk, neck and arms, particularly on the more affected side; B. Hemidyskinesia with arm-greater-than leg involvement can also be a manifestation of peak-dose dyskinesias, especially among young-onset PD patients; C. Diphasic dyskinesias predominantly affect the legs, while relatively sparing the trunk, neck, and arms; D. Unilateral foot dystonia on the more affected side is the typical manifestation of "off" dystonia; E. Facial choreathetotic movements and hand posturing may occur in advanced PD patients; F. Facial dystonia with feet dyskinesias are a topographical distribution atypical for PD and suggestive of multiple system atrophy. Darker gray emphasizes greater severity. (Figure by Martha Headworth, University of Cincinnati Neuroscience Institute. Adapted with permission from Espay 2010[18].)

response to subthalamic nucleus deep brain stimulation, suggesting that they are manifestations of different activity patterns in the subthalamic nucleus or downstream structures.[17] These motor phenomena are pharmacodynamic complications aggravated by pharmacokinetic liabilities, particularly the short half-life of L-dopa and incomplete or unreliable levodopa absorption in the duodenum. Other dyskinetic patterns are illustrated in Figure 6.4D–F. In more advanced PD, dyskinesias may become more prominent in the face while lessening in the limbs. Beware of the dyskinesia pattern involving dystonia of the lower face and chorea of the feet early in the course of parkinsonism (Figure 6.4F). This pattern of L-dopa-induced dyskinesia is more typical of multiple system atrophy.

Diagnosis: Diphasic dyskinesia in a patient with PD

Tip: *Lower body predominant dyskinesias are treated by increasing rather than decreasing the stimulation of dopamine receptors.*

Case 33: Feet twisting after walking

Case: This 38-year-old woman had a 4-year history of plantar flexion and eversion of the left foot that developed only after walking briskly on a treadmill for 45 minutes. Her symptoms would resolve with rest. Over time, however, the latency to foot posturing would decrease such that only 25 minutes of walking were sufficient to bring it on and longer periods of rest were needed to restore baseline (Video 33).

What pattern could be missed in this case?

The induction by exercise distinguishes this form of dystonia from other forms of primary dystonia. Lacking this specific inductor (exercise), one would have to suspect a lesion in the contralateral basal ganglia, since adult-onset dystonia in the feet is extremely rare in primary dystonias. This case presentation is classical for paroxysmal exercise-induced dystonia (PED) but can be overlooked or misdiagnosed as psychogenic.

If we had access to one test and one treatment, which would they be?

In PED, the diagnostic test of choice is the evaluation on CSF of dopamine and serotonin metabolism. A treatment trial with L-dopa, after CSF has been collected and interpreted, would be the critical treatment strategy. Although PED is often idiopathic, it can be the presenting manifestation of dopa-responsive dystonia (DRD) or can antedate the onset of PD by many years. In either situation, a low homovanillic acid in CSF is likely, with or without other abnormalities that may help localize the affected enzymatic pathway in the case of DRD. Where available, a DAT SPECT scan can be particularly useful in differentiating young-onset PD from DRD, as it is likely to be abnormal in the former but normal in the latter.[20]

Besides a low HVA, there were no other abnormalities in the CSF. The patient refused treatment. However, 3 years later she developed tremor, bradykinesia, and rigidity in the same side as her foot dystonia. She had an excellent response to treatment with pramipexole 3 mg/day.

Discussion: Although dystonic symptoms are common in the setting of PD, they do not commonly predate the disease. In fully established PD, dystonic symptoms tend to represent wearing off of L-dopa. In untreated PD, dystonia at presentation may be more common among those with onset below 40 years (early-onset PD, EOPD). Foot dystonia is the presenting feature in 42% of patients with autosomal recessive-juvenile parkinsonism (AR-JP), particularly due to the *Parkin* gene, although most patients do not have the PED phenotype.[21] When PED is the harbinger for PD, the threshold of exercise required to elicit dystonia progressively lowers and eventually the parkinsonian features become constantly present in the same side affected by PED.[22] This patient's PED may be considered the earliest feature of the otherwise classic PD that followed.

The diagnostic implications for PED have grown and the idiopathic category is likely to be reduced further over time. In addition to DRD (particularly due to GTP cyclohydrolase 1 deficiency or tyrosine hydroxylase deficiency) and PD, another etiology to consider in PED, especially if epilepsy is part of the clinical picture, is glucose transport protein type 1 (GLUT1) deficiency syndrome due to mutations in the *SLC2A1* gene, associated with low CSF glucose and treated with a ketogenic diet.[23]

Diagnosis: Paroxysmal exercise-induced dystonia antedating PD

Tip: *PED can antedate PD by many years or be the presenting phenotype of DRD or GLUT1 deficiency syndrome. CSF studies offer critical clues in this ostensibly benign dystonic phenotype.*

Case 34: Anxiety and shortness of breath in PD

Case: This 50-year-old woman had symptoms consistent with PD for 6 years. She had been well controlled with ropinirole first, and L-dopa added later. Her tremor had all but disappeared and she claimed only mild foot cramping and twisting in the mornings and intermittently throughout the day. She admitted to no motor fluctuations. Over the last year, however, she had experienced random episodes of anxiety with palpitations, shortness of breath, hyperventilation, and occasionally chest pain. She had undergone extensive cardiovascular and respiratory investigations over the course of two separate emergency department visits but no abnormalities had been uncovered. Lorazepam had been prescribed for as-needed use.

What is the major pitfall in this case?

Lack of overt motor fluctuations does not imply absence of non-motor fluctuations. The only evidence of wearing off may be in the non-motor sphere, whereby there is no concurrent re-emergence of tremor, gait impairment, or other motor features. In this case, the clinician failed to acknowledge the possibility that cardiorespiratory features more likely represented L-dopa wearing off. The pattern

of "random" episodes of anxiety is often overlooked and mistreated as unrelated to the disease and its treatment. In fact, the addition of entacapone, a catechol-*O*-methyl transferase (COMT)-inhibitor, eliminated all symptoms of anxiety and shortness of breath, and the need for lorazepam.

Discussion: Non-motor fluctuations can present in a variety of subtle ways, easily overlooked by the motor-centric view of the Parkinson's world (for another wrinkle on this theme, see Case 11). Anxiety and panic attacks are among the most disabling as well as under- and mistreated symptoms in PD. It is surprising, then, that these symptoms should be responsive to simple strategies aimed at increasing the dopaminergic tone.[24] While off-period anxiety, apathy, and fatigue occur in up to 75% of patients,[25] history alone may not confirm a relationship with dosing cycles, emphasizing the importance of at least suspecting their relationship with "off" and "on" periods. This is critical when considering that almost a third of patients with PD derive greater disability from non-motor than from motor fluctuations.[25] In difficult cases, an acute apomorphine challenge can be used in a similar manner to the "Tensilon test" in myasthenia gravis, to help determine whether a given clinical feature represents over- or under-stimulation of central dopamine receptors.[26] In many centers it is easier to simply observe patients through the course of a L-dopa dose challenge (an "off-on" study). Patients come into the clinic after an overnight drug withdrawal, at least 12 hours after the last dopaminergic dose, in the so-called practically defined "off" period. They then receive their usual or a supramaximal dose of L-dopa to ensure a definite "switch on." Motor and non-motor phenomena can be thus appreciated and documented in the corresponding treatment period.

Inasmuch as these fluctuations can be a reflection of the short half-life of L-dopa, mechanisms to minimize its pharmacokinetic peaks and troughs should include methods to extend L-dopa's duration of action through changes in the dose or dosing schedule, or by adding a COMT inhibitor, a MAO-B inhibitor, or a dopamine agonist in young, cognitively

Table 6.3. Selected L-dopa-responsive and non-L-dopa-responsive motor and non-motor fluctuations

L-dopa-responsive fluctuations		L-dopa-unresponsive fluctuations	
Motor	Non-motor	Motor	Non-motor
Tremor	Anxiety	Falls	Apathy, anhedonia
Bradykinesia	Panic attacks	Freezing of gait	Hallucinations
Rigidity	Paroxysmal sweating	Postural instability	Orthostatic hypotension
Gait impairment	Pain	Speech impairment	Depression
Dyskinesias	Hallucinations		Constipation
	Confusion		Erectile dysfunction
	Fatigue		Dysphagia
	Numbness/tingling		Drooling
	Restless leg syndrome		

intact individuals. Anxiety, pain, fatigue, and sensory symptoms are among the non-motor fluctuations that could inappropriately prompt clinicians to consider symptomatic therapies (anxiolytics, analgesics, etc.) when fine tuning the dopaminergic treatment would have sufficed. However, not all non-motor fluctuations are L-dopa responsive (Table 6.3).[27]

A cautionary tale regarding the connection between mood and L-dopa is worth keeping in mind. When patients appreciate the connection between mood elevation and L-dopa, they may increase their L-dopa dose in order to reach a hypomanic or true manic state, often also rendering them severely dyskinetic. This addictive behavior falls under the umbrella of the "dopamine dysregulation syndrome" (DDS).[28] These patients may also display hypersexuality, pathological gambling, and compulsive shopping or eating, although these impulse control disorders (ICDs) are more commonly complications of dopamine agonist treatment and not necessarily representative of DDS, which is seen with shorter acting drugs such as L-dopa and apomorphine. In addition, patients may engage in repetitive, meaningless, seemingly purposeless tasks or stereotypical behaviors termed "punding."[29] These behaviors occur at the expense of sleep, and take place over many hours every day. A milder form of this is "hobbyism," where patients spend excessive amounts of time engrossed in more purposeful activities, such as painting, woodwork, etc.[19]

Diagnosis: Anxiety as dopaminergic wearing off in PD

Tip: *Before embarking on complex tests or treatments for autonomic, sensory, cognitive, or behavioral symptoms in PD, consider adjustments in the dose of dopaminergic drugs, as these problems more often represent non-motor fluctuations.*

Case 35: Unusual tics in "Tourette syndrome"

Contributed by Dr. Don Gilbert, Cincinnati, Ohio

Case: This 17-year-old female high school student developed sudden onset of head jerking while sitting with a peer group reflecting quietly on an upcoming international trip. Jerking occurred constantly while awake. She reported the movements were involuntary, not accompanied by premonitory urge, and not suppressible. On examination, there was repetitive and patterned neck jerking, but close observation showed some variability in head and chin direction (Video 35).

What are the main holes that can be drilled into this case of "Tourette syndrome"?

First, after observing the jerks for a couple of minutes, it becomes clear the movements are not exactly stereotypical: subtle and overt variability

Table 6.4. Features in Tourette syndrome and psychogenic tourettism

Tourette features	Features of Tourette *and* pseudo-tics	Pseudo-tics features
Premonitory urge	Abrupt onset	Maximum disability at onset
Suppressibility	Cessation with distraction	Increase with attention
Appreciated as partially voluntary	Response to placebo or suggestion	Variability between tics
Relief in performing movement	Waxing and waning course	Frequency of tics may be entrained
	Dramatic resolution	

emerges between them. Second, they do not follow the rule of disappearing during voluntary movements that is typical for the motor and vocal tics in Tourette syndrome. This "suppressibility" during activity and re-emergence while at rest is typical of Tourette syndrome, which provides an example where this feature does not imply psychogenicity. In fact, the lack of premonitory urge and suppressibility in "Tourette" tics is most suggestive of pseudo-tics and should prepare the clinician to hunt for other psychogenic features and the potential stressors feeding into this psychogenic phenotype.[30]

One must be mindful, therefore, that a number of the criteria used to define psychogenic movement disorders, particularly those originally described for psychogenic dystonia,[31] do not necessarily distinguish organic Tourette syndrome from psychogenic tourettism (Table 6.4). The strict application of these criteria may falsely classify Tourette syndrome as psychogenic.[32]

Discussion: The repeated simple or complex motor tics in Tourette syndrome should be nearly identical to one another. These perfectly patterned repetitive movements define the classic stereotypic nature of tics in this disorder. It is important to note that the behavioral accompaniments of tics are helpful in supporting or, as this case demonstrates, excluding the diagnosis of Tourette syndrome. This patient did not acknowledge an urge prior to the tics, a subjective relief following each of them, or any ability to suppress the movements transiently. These features are almost never absent in Tourette syndrome. The latter clinical feature, in particular, is also followed by a need to "release" the tics

during moments of rising stress.[33] The entrainment of this patient's jerks during various tasks and their persistence (and even enhancement) during finger-to-nose and walking tasks were icing on the cake in the diagnosis of pseudo-tics, which should have become clear upon recognizing this pattern in the first 30 seconds of the exam.

Diagnosis: Pseudo-tics (psychogenic tourettism)

Tip: *It is important to differentiate pseudo-tics from organic tics in children with Tourette syndrome in order to initiate appropriate behavioral treatments rather than potentially harmful pharmacotherapy.*

REFERENCES

1. Beric A, Kelly PJ, Rezai A, et al. Complications of deep brain stimulation surgery. *Stereotact Funct Neurosurg* 2001;**77**(1–4):73–78.
2. Miranda M, Chana P. Severe off-period facial dystonia in Parkinson's disease. *Mov Disord* 2000;**15**(1):163–164.
3. Wenning GK, Geser F, Poewe W. The 'risus sardonicus' of multiple system atrophy. *Mov Disord* 2003;**18**(10):1211.
4. Wenning GK, Quinn NP, Daniel SE, et al. Facial dystonia in pathologically proven multiple system atrophy: a video report. *Mov Disord* 1996;**11**(1):107–109.
5. Schrag A, Munchau A, Bhatia KP, et al. Essential tremor: an overdiagnosed condition? *J Neurol* 2000;**247**(12):955–959.
6. Jain S, Lo SE, Louis ED. Common misdiagnosis of a common neurological disorder: how are we misdiagnosing essential tremor? *Arch Neurol* 2006;**63**(8):1100–1104.
7. Jedynak CP, Bonnet AM, Agid Y. Tremor and idiopathic dystonia. *Mov Disord* 1991;**6**(3):230–236.
8. Heroux ME, Pari G, Norman KE. The effect of inertial loading on wrist postural tremor in essential tremor. *Clin Neurophysiol* 2009;**120**(5):1020–1029.

9. Lang AE, Jog M, Ashby P. "Weight-holding tremor": an unusual task-specific form of essential tremor? *Mov Disord* 1995;**10**(2):228–229.

10. Schwartz MA, Selhorst JB, Ochs AL, et al. Oculomasticatory myorhythmia: a unique movement disorder occurring in Whipple's disease. *Ann Neurol* 1986;**20**(6):677–683.

11. Louis ED, Lynch T, Kaufmann P, et al. Diagnostic guidelines in central nervous system Whipple's disease. *Ann Neurol* 1996;**40**(4):561–568.

12. Masucci EF, Kurtzke JF, Saini N. Myorhythmia: a widespread movement disorder. Clinicopathological correlations. *Brain* 1984;**107** (Pt 1):53–79.

13. Deuschl G, Toro C, Valls-Sole J, et al. Symptomatic and essential palatal tremor. 1. Clinical, physiological and MRI analysis. *Brain* 1994;**117** (Pt 4):775–788.

14. Revilla FJ, de la Cruz R, Khardori N, et al. Teaching NeuroImage: oculomasticatory myorhythmia: pathognomonic phenomenology of Whipple disease. *Neurology* 2008;**70**(6):e25.

15. Fahn S. The spectrum of levodopa-induced dyskinesias. *Ann Neurol* 2000;**47**(4 Suppl 1):S2–S9.

16. Jankovic J. Motor fluctuations and dyskinesias in Parkinson's disease: clinical manifestations. *Mov Disord* 2005;**20** Suppl 11:S11–S16.

17. Krack P, Pollak P, Limousin P, et al. From off-period dystonia to peak-dose chorea: the clinical spectrum of varying subthalamic nucleus activity. *Brain* 1999;**122** (Pt 6):1133–1146.

18. Espay AJ. Management of motor complications in Parkinson disease: current and emerging therapies. *Neurol Clin* 2010;**28**(4):913–925.

19. Fox SH, Lang AE. Levodopa-related motor complications – phenomenology. *Mov Disord* 2008;**23** Suppl 3:S509–S514.

20. Katzenschlager R, Costa D, Gacinovic S, et al. [(123)I]-FP-CIT-SPECT in the early diagnosis of PD presenting as exercise-induced dystonia. *Neurology* 2002;**59**(12):1974–1976.

21. Khan NL, Graham E, Critchley P, et al. Parkin disease: a phenotypic study of a large case series. *Brain* 2003;**126** (Pt 6):1279–1292.

22. Bozi M, Bhatia KP. Paroxysmal exercise-induced dystonia as a presenting feature of young-onset Parkinson's disease. *Mov Disord* 2003;**18**(12):1545–1547.

23. Brockmann K. The expanding phenotype of GLUT1-deficiency syndrome. *Brain Dev* 2009;**31**(7):545–552.

24. Khan W, Naz S, Rana AQ. Shortness of breath, a 'wearing-off' symptom in Parkinson's disease. *Clin Drug Investig* 2009;**29**(10):689–691.

25. Witjas T, Kaphan E, Azulay JP, et al. Nonmotor fluctuations in Parkinson's disease: frequent and disabling. *Neurology* 2002;**59**(3):408–413.

26. Quinn NP. Classification of fluctuations in patients with Parkinson's disease. *Neurology* 1998;**51**(2 Suppl 2):S25–S29.

27. Riley DE, Lang AE. The spectrum of levodopa-related fluctuations in Parkinson's disease. *Neurology* 1993;**43**(8):1459–1464.

28. Lawrence AD, Evans AH, Lees AJ. Compulsive use of dopamine replacement therapy in Parkinson's disease: reward systems gone awry? *Lancet Neurol* 2003;**2**(10):595–604.

29. Evans AH, Katzenschlager R, Paviour D, et al. Punding in Parkinson's disease: its relation to the dopamine dysregulation syndrome. *Mov Disord* 2004;**19**(4):397–405.

30. Kurlan R, Deeley C, Como PG. Psychogenic movement disorder (pseudo-tics) in a patient with Tourette's syndrome. *J Neuropsychiatry Clin Neurosci* 1992;**4**(3):347–348.

31. Fahn S, Williams DT. Psychogenic dystonia. *Adv Neurol* 1988;**50**:431–455.

32. Mejia NI, Jankovic J. Secondary tics and tourettism. *Rev Bras Psiquiatr* 2005;**27**(1):11–17.

33. Dooley JM, Stokes A, Gordon KE. Pseudo-tics in Tourette syndrome. *J Child Neurol* 1994;**9**(1):50–51.

7

Testing pitfalls of commission or omission

Case 36: Low HVA and BH$_4$ in "DRD"

With the contribution of Dr. Leo Verhagen, Chicago, Illinois

Case: This 20-year-old woman developed progressive resting and action tremor in both hands at the age of 13 years. Stiffness, slowness, and mild difficulty with balance followed. Her speech became softer and slurred and her handwriting micrographic. At age 14 she was started on L-dopa with excellent response. However, within 6 months of L-dopa therapy she developed wearing off fluctuations and severe peak-dose dyskinesias, despite low doses (50 mg thrice daily). Amantadine paradoxically worsened them and was discontinued within days. Her mother noticed occasional brief episodes where she would look up involuntarily. By age 15, her school performance decreased and an uncharacteristic pattern of lower school grades were reported. Episodes of agitation and lack of judgment became important problems and she endorsed feelings of depression and crying spells. On examination, she was noted to have end-gaze nystagmus with a full range of ocular motion, though she had to blink and move her head to initiate saccades. The voice was hypophonic and labored. Rigidity and hypokinesia were prominent in the "off" state. Dystonic and choreoathetotic movements were present in her face, tongue, and hands in the "on" state (Video 36). Neuropsychological testing revealed average intellectual abilities but significant weakness in memory and executive function.

How can we be led astray with the testing?

By relying on the CSF dopamine metabolites for a patient whose parkinsonian phenotype of early onset and marked responsiveness to L-dopa makes one highly suspicious of dopa-responsive dystonia (DRD) or a genetic form of PD. Indeed, homovanillic acid (HVA) (71 [normal, 167–563]) and tetrahydrobiopterin (BH$_4$) (8 [9–32]) were low while 5-HIAA, 3-O-methyldopa, and neopterin were normal. On the other hand, her F-DOPA PET demonstrated symmetrically decreased uptake in the putamen and, to a lesser extent, caudate bilaterally. Testing was unremarkable for ceruloplasmin, serum copper, vitamin B$_{12}$, folate, and coenzyme Q10.

Shouldn't low HVA and BH$_4$ suffice for the diagnosis of DRD?

Though the case for DRD was buttressed by the findings of low HVA and BH$_4$ in a young parkinsonian woman markedly responsive to L-dopa and possibly experiencing oculogyric crisis, the evidence against DRD was more compelling. First, motor fluctuations with prominent dyskinesias are features of nigral degenerative processes such as PD, particularly due to mutations in the *Parkin* gene. DRD is not associated with nigral degeneration; hence, motor fluctuations and dyskinesias should not be part of the clinical spectrum. In this patient, the unusual distribution of dyskinesias would make a parkinsonism other than PD more likely. Second, the progressive cognitive and

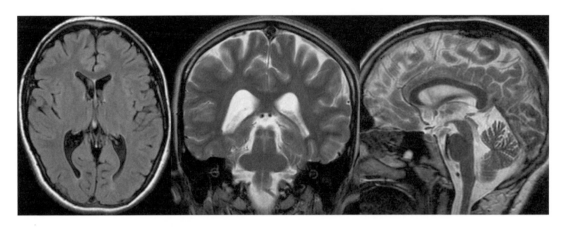

Figure 7.1. Axial FLAIR, coronal T2- and mid-sagittal T2-weighted brain MRI showing mild but definite cortical and subcortical brain and cerebellar atrophy. Patient was 15 years old.

behavioral changes, especially early in the disease course, strongly argued against the diagnosis. Third, F-DOPA PET should be normal in DRD. The CSF profile suggested the dominant form of DRD due to mutations in the GTP cyclohydrolase 1 gene but excluded the autosomal recessive causes of the DRD syndrome, tyrosine hydroxylase (TH) and sepiapterin reductase (SR) deficiencies.

Genetic testing was negative for mutations in the GTP cyclohydrolase 1 gene. Also there were no mutations/expansions in the *Parkin* gene, IT15, and ataxin-3. The brain MRI showed mild atrophy (Figure 7.1). EEG showed abnormal, generalized epileptiform discharges with intermixed 1–2 second high voltage slow waves with no clinical correlation and no electrographic seizures. Prolonged EEG monitoring showed bursts of bifrontal-predominant, spike-and-wave epileptiform activity, not increasing in frequency during sleep. Motor and sensory nerve conduction studies were normal. EMG needle examination of the left leg showed large motor unit action potentials with prolonged duration, suggestive of chronic reinnervation with no active denervation, consistent with axonal neuropathy. Muscle biopsy showed a general loss of the normal mosaic pattern of fiber-type grouping, interpreted as active chronic neuropathic changes, typical of lower motor neuron disorders.

What is the diagnostic test of choice?

The patient declined a full-thickness rectal biopsy, the usual test of choice for the suspected diagnosis. However, her interest and her family's in proceeding with deep brain stimulation to improve her parkinsonism and motor fluctuations provided an opportunity to obtain cerebral tissue during the procedure. The brain biopsy was diagnostic of neuronal intranuclear inclusion disease (NIID), a rare sporadic disorder often associated with L-dopa-responsive juvenile parkinsonism. Additional neurological involvement in NIID includes cognitive and behavioral disturbances, motor neuropathy, and particularly oculogyric crises.[1] Pathological diagnosis can be made ante-mortem on full-thickness rectal biopsy with intranuclear inclusions and neuronal death in the myenteric plexus.

Discussion: Although most adults with atypical parkinsonism are poorly L-dopa responsive, three conditions exhibit marked levodopa responsiveness in juvenile-onset disease (< 20 years): *Parkin* mutations (autosomal recessive, most common), DRD (mostly autosomal dominant, rare), and NIID (usually sporadic, very rare).[2] A short list of other conditions must be kept in mind in cases of L-dopa-responsive early-onset atypical parkinsonism

Table 7.1. L-dopa-responsive juvenile or early-onset parkinsonisms

Nomenclature	Disorder and inheritance
DYT5a	AD – Dopa-responsive dystonia due to *GCH1* mutations
DYT5b	AR – Dopa-responsive dystonia due to *TH* mutations or sepiapterin reductase deficiency
DYT16	AR – Dystonia-parkinsonism due to *PRKRA* mutations
SCA3*	AD – Spinocerebellar ataxia type 3
PARK2	AR – *Parkin* disease
PARK6	AR – PINK1-associated PD
PARK7	AR – DJ1-associated PD
PARK9	AR – Kufor-Rakeb disease
PARK14	AR – *PLA2G6*-associated neurodegeneration (PLAN)
SPG11	AR – Hereditary spastic paraparesis with thin corpus callosum
PKAN	AR – Pantothenate kinase-associated neurodegeneration (neurodegeneration with brain iron accumulation 1 [NBIA1])
NIID	Sporadic – neuronal intranuclear inclusion disease (this case)

* SCA2 can also present with L-dopa-responsive parkinsonism but ataxia and slowed saccades tend to dominate the clinical picture. AR, autosomal recessive inheritance; AD, autosomal dominant inheritance.

(Table 7.1). This patient's striking response to levodopa, presence of oculogyric crises, and decreased HVA and BH$_4$ were compelling for DRD. However, the parkinsonian phenotype of DRD typically begins in adulthood, dyskinesias are uncommon (never reported in the facial region), the motor response to levodopa is sustained, and tremor may remain prominent throughout the disease.[3] The abnormal F-dopa PET study decisively ruled DRD out.

During the diagnostic efforts, the clinicians involved in the care of this patient found support in their migration from a diagnosis of DRD to NIID from a similar juvenile parkinsonian case first reported as "DRD with Lewy bodies."[4] As in the present case, that report described marked

levodopa responsiveness, oculogyric crises, and decreased HVA in CSF.[5] A shrewd group of neurologists, keenly aware of the rarity of Lewy bodies in juvenile parkinsonism, re-examined the pathology of the case over a decade later and determined that the eosinophilic and ubiquitinated inclusions were actually intranuclear, indeed revising the diagnosis to NIID.[6] NIID more typically presents in the first two decades of life as multisystem degeneration with pyramidal, extrapyramidal, and cerebellar signs, as well as behavioral and cognitive disturbances. Parkinsonism (L-dopa responsive or resistant) has been the predominant clinical feature in a handful of previously reported NIID cases. Clearly, low HVA and BH$_4$ were red herrings in a story that could not easily fit into the DRD pigeonhole.

Diagnosis: Neuronal intranuclear inclusion disease

Tip: *A CSF profile consistent with "dopa-responsive dystonia" may hide neuronal intranuclear inclusion disease or other L-dopa-responsive juvenile or early-onset parkinsonian disorders. A recent report suggests that skin biopsy may effectively replace rectal biopsy in the diagnosis of NIID.*

Case 37: Potential for over-testing in ataxia

Case: This 52-year-old woman had variable degrees of balance impairment, weakness, and clumsiness for about 5 years. She progressed to the point of being barely able to stand and take steps without assistance, and she became confined to a wheelchair. She developed a right foot drop. She felt clumsy in her hands and her handwriting became large and chaotic. She had chronic diarrhea since the onset of her problems. She also reported that liquids may go up through her nose and admitted to urinary incontinence, excessive sweating when exposed to heat, cataracts diagnosed in her mid 40s, and dry eyes. Examination showed a distal-to-proximal gradient of weakness in the legs to a greater extent than the arms, areflexia, truncal and appendicular ataxia, and impaired sensation to all sensory modalities, though position sense was affected to a lesser extent than temperature, touch, and vibration. She had a severe waddling, wide-based gait (Video 37).

For this ataxic syndrome, the plan was decidedly unassertive. The initial testing included a range of disparate tests including antigliadin antibodies for celiac disease, basic rheumatologic panel, serum copper and ceruloplasmin, and the intention to examine for paraneoplastic cerebellar ataxia (she had accumulated a 31 pack/year history of cigarette smoking), particularly in view of her severe peripheral neuropathy.

How can the characterization of this ataxic syndrome help in the diagnostic process?

Though dysmetria was prominent, especially in the legs, leg weakness was the dominant feature and it, alone, could have explained the clumsiness. Her wide base of support and need for assistance to stand and take steps made it impossible to test for Romberg sign, which would certainly have been present. Very importantly, a leg-predominant pattern of weakness with distal loss of pain, temperature, vibration, and, to a lesser extent, joint position sense should have certainly suggested demyelinating peripheral neuropathy as accounting for at least some (if not all) of the ataxic syndrome.

How to simplify testing?

High-yield testing can be orchestrated by focusing on the most severe manifestation: the peripheral neuropathic process. Indeed, a sural nerve biopsy confirmed a demyelinating rather than axonal neuropathy and, with that lead, testing was positive for IgM antibodies to myelin-associated glycoprotein (MAG), with titers twice the upper limit of normal. A diagnosis of IgM-MGUS neuropathy was made. Prior neuroimaging had shown normal spinal cord signal and bulk. There was relatively mild vermal cerebellar atrophy (which explained the hypermetric saccades, the only oculomotor findings) but otherwise normal cerebellum.

Discussion: If the loss of position sense were to have been greater than the loss of other sensory modalities, then a posterior column myelopathy and a sensory neuronopathy or ganglionopathy would be the categories worth pursuing for testing (see Table 5.1). Instead, as the pattern of sensory deprivation favored temperature and vibration over position sense, and weakness was part of the phenotype, the immune-mediated *demyelinating* sensorimotor peripheral neuropathies or polyradiculopathies should have come to the fore at the earliest evaluation. Within this category, there are three main conditions to consider (with the corresponding testing): the Miller Fisher variant of Guillain-Barré syndrome (anti-GQ1b), the sensory ataxic neuropathy (anti-GD1b), and the anti-MAG neuropathy (MAG-SGPG). The first two, typically acute, appear to form part of a clinical continuum.[7] Apparently the proprioceptive nerves can barely tell apart the "Q" in GQ1b from the "D" in GD1b and such features as albuminocytological dissociation, preceding infectious symptoms, and distal paraesthesias occur just as frequently in both conditions. In contrast, this patient had a slowly progressive truncal and lower appendicular ataxia with demyelinating *sensorimotor* polyneuropathy that is common among those with IgM monoclonal gammopathy of unknown significance (MGUS) with IgM antibodies against MAG or sulfoglucuronyl paragloboside (SGPG).

MGUS neuropathy comprises 60% of all paraproteinemias and has been reported to occur in up to 3% of people over the age of 50 years. Associated with MAG antibodies in over 50% of cases, it expresses as a painless, slowly progressive, large-fiber neuropathy. The clinical picture may include sensory ataxia, tremor, and leg weakness and the conduction velocity studies show demyelinating features, though secondary axonal loss ultimately occurs.[8] Plasma exchange has been suggested as a line of treatment for severe cases, followed by a regimen of monthly pulses with prednisone and cyclophosphamide or rituximab.[9] Other polyneuropathies associated with paraproteinemias include (1) distal acquired demyelinating symmetric (DADS-M) neuropathy, which is best known as the ataxic, sensory predominant CIDP variant; (2) neuropathy associated with primary systemic amyloidosis, which is accompanied by autonomic dysfunction; (3) neuropathy of polyneuropathy, organomegaly, endocrinopathy, M protein, and skin changes (POEMS) syndrome; and (4) neuropathy associated with Waldenström macroglobulinemia. Anti-MAG antibodies play a causative role in IgM-MGUS, DADS-M, and Waldenström's macroglobulinemia. The latter is axonal (as in primary systemic amyloidosis), the first two demyelinating (as in POEMS). Sensory ataxia can be a prominent feature of these three anti-MAG-IgM associated *demyelinating* polyneuropathies, and as such may be considered part of the same spectrum of polyneuropathies.[10]

Diagnosis: IgM-MGUS neuropathy associated with MAG antibodies

Tip: *Ataxia with weakness and sensory loss should focus testing on the demyelinating peripheral neuropathies. Sensory ataxias may mistakenly be worked up as cerebellar ataxias.*

Case 38: "Variant of unknown significance" in genetic testing of PD

Case: This 52-year-old woman developed pain in the left shoulder and arm tightness about 20 years prior to this evaluation. Left-hand resting tremor appeared 12 years later and abated completely after initiation of L-dopa treatment. However, this treatment made her "jerky" in the left arm and brought out some "restlessness" in the left leg, which did not affect her walking. Over time, she noted that as each L-dopa dose would wear off she became restless and anxious, sometimes needing to pace about (reported by patient in Video 38). There was no family history of PD.

Are there guidelines for testing this patient?

She fits within the construct of early-onset Parkinson's disease (EOPD) by virtue of a disease onset younger than 40 years of age. Generally, the

Table 7.2. Clinical features of mutation carriers

Feature	More common in mutation carriers vs. non-carriers
Age	Younger (for AR forms; not necessarily for AD *LRRK2*)
Sidedness	More symmetrical presentation
Initial sign	Dystonia as an initial sign
	Hyperreflexia as examination feature
Progression	Slower disease progression
Response to treatment	Excellent and sustained response to levodopa treatment with early development of motor and non-motor complications

Although these features have been formally ascertained only for *Parkin* mutation carriers compared with matched patients without *Parkin* mutations, they represent clinical clues for genetic PD in general.

younger the age of onset, the more frequent a monogenic origin of PD, and the more sensible it is to pursue genetic tests. The clinical picture is highly suggestive of EOPD: rapid response to L-dopa at introductory doses with prompt development of motor and non-motor complications (Table 7.2). Dystonia with non-motor "off state" symptoms of painful shoulder and anxiety are typical presentations of PD among those in the younger age bracket. Pain, in particular, seems more often reported in the context of PD patients with the autosomal recessive *PINK1* mutations (see Cases 3 and 4 in Klein's review[11]) and the autosomal dominant LRRK2 mutations (Klein's Case 6[11]). Besides the clinical picture, age and family history are important guidelines for testing (Table 7.3), taking into account that family history may be "pseudo-negative" in such situations as small families, non-paternity, adoption, variable expressivity, reduced penetrance, or de novo mutations. Despite a negative family history, which may have indeed been pseudo-negative, this case was similar to Klein's Case 4 (due to a homozygous mutation in *PINK1*), with parallels including an earlier suspicion that this patient had a form of conversion disorder. Genetic testing for *Parkin* and *PINK1* was pursued.

Table 7.3. Suggested genetic testing guidelines for PD

Family history	Juvenile PD (< 20 years)	EOPD (20–40 years)	Adult (> 40 years)
Positive	Recessive genes: *Parkin, PINK1, DJ1*	Recessive genes: *Parkin, PINK1, DJ1* Dominant genes: *LRRK2, SNCA, GCH1*	Dominant genes: *LRRK2, SNCA* Recessive genes: *Parkin, PINK1, DJ1*
Negative	Recessive genes: *Parkin, PINK1, DJ1*	Mutations rarely found	Mutations rarely found

GCH1: GTP cyclohydrolase I; *LRRK2*: leucine-rich repeat kinase 2; *PINK1*, PTEN-induced putative kinase 1; *SNCA*: α-synuclein. EOPD: early-onset Parkinson's disease.
As suggested by Klein.[11]

Genetic testing (Athena Diagnostics) in this patient demonstrated two variants in exon 10 and 11 of the *Parkin* gene that represented known polymorphisms, as well as a "variant of unknown significance" in codon 115 of the *PINK1* gene. The latter could be causative (unknown significance means that studies in large families with this particular genetic endowment have not been carried out to determine whether it can be truly pathogenic) or could represent a genetic susceptibility explaining a picture of parkinsonism and dystonic pain previously reported within the genetic spectrum of *PINK1* gene mutations.

Discussion: PD-related gene mutations range from clearly pathogenic (e.g., a homozygous mutation in a fully penetrant recessive disorder) to those associated with an increased risk (e.g., heterozygous GBA mutations).[12] *Parkin* mutations account for about 60% of patients with disease onset before the age of 30 years. *PINK1* (*PTEN*-induced putative kinase 1) mutations are the second most common cause of EOPD with a mutation frequency ranging from 1% to 9%.[13] Four of the known genetic mutations causing PD, *Parkin, PINK1, DJ1*, and LRRK2, only account for about 1% of all cases of PD, only 20% of early-onset PD, and less than 3% of late-onset PD at best.[11] Testing guidelines have been suggested for PD according to family history (sporadic vs. familial; recessive vs. dominant), and age at onset (juvenile, early-onset, and late-onset) (Table 7.3). Dystonia and pain (or other non-motor

features) can be prominent in some hereditary forms of PD. In fact, a form of late-onset L-dopa-responsive dystonia owing to mutations in the *GCH1* gene may rarely present as PD.

Although genetic testing does not necessarily alter management and can be costly, it is important to consider in selected cases for genetic counseling, to estimate rate of progression, and to raise alertness for common motor and behavioral complications related to treatment. Although the individual clinical course cannot be predicted, the general rule is that patients with genetic PD have a more slowly progressive condition, respond better to treatment, and develop fewer of the motor disabilities than patients without these mutations. In addition, the autosomal recessive forms typically have much less dysautonomia and cognitive changes. In the future, patients with genetic premotor PD and mutation carriers at risk may be critical for evaluating neuroprotective treatment strategies.

Of parenthetical interest, pain is the most common complaint that brings patients to physicians other than neurologists, with frozen shoulder being the most common related misdiagnosis in PD.[14] Most pain-ridden patients also happen to lack early tremor, rigidity, and bradykinesia, further delaying the diagnosis, as was illustrated in this case.[14] Shoulder or proximal arm pain, often with features of a frozen shoulder, is not uncommon as a presenting feature in PD and can lead to a variety of misdiagnoses (and unnecessary invasive procedures) such as bursitis, rotator cuff injury, tendonitis, frozen shoulder from other causes, and other orthopedic or arthritic conditions.[15] The shoulder discomfort obviously persists until appropriate anti-PD pharmacotherapy is initiated.

Diagnosis: Early-onset PD associated with a variant in the *PINK1* gene of unknown significance

Tip: *In early-onset PD with excellent response and rapid development of motor (e.g., dyskinesias) and/or behavioral complications (e.g., anxiety) after introductory doses of L-dopa, a genetic parkinsonism is likely, whether the commercially available genetic testing confirms it, refutes it, or is of "unknown significance."*

Case 39: Multiple positive results in chorea: perils of the shot-gun approach

Case: This 72-year-old woman had rocking head movements for about 6 years prior to her evaluation. Partial complex seizures with post-ictal confusion and separate syncopal episodes due to atrioventricular nodal re-entry tachycardia had emerged 2.5 years ago. Treatment with levetiracetam and AV nodal ablation eliminated the seizures and syncope. For the prior 6 months, she exhibited throat clearing movements that she could voluntarily withhold, were preceded by mild urge, and were partly relieved by each movement (Video 39). She also felt clumsy handling utensils or pouring water or coffee and admitted to forgetfulness. She had a history of depression, rheumatoid arthritis, and hypothyroidism.

Did the examination findings allow focused testing?

The patient demonstrated facial, cervical, and bilateral arm chorea with tic-like movements, proximal leg weakness, arreflexia, mild truncal ataxia, and peripheral neuropathy. Her cognitive screen was normal (MMSE = 30/30; Frontal Assessment Battery = 18/18). The combination of seizures, arreflexia, myopathic weakness, and peripheral neuropathy favored chorea-acanthocytosis. Seizures can also be present in spinocerebellar ataxia type 17 (SCA 17), a rare adult-onset form of chorea. Finally, other important causes of chorea are antiphospholipid antibody syndrome, celiac disease, and Huntington's disease. The latter was felt highly unlikely given the lack of family history, normal cognitive screen, and absence of oculomotor apraxia or tongue protrusion impersistence. Hence, besides HD, there were a disparate group of conditions potentially explaining this patient's deficits. A major pitfall is to test for all these conditions at once without a sense of priority.

What single test would have helped most in prioritizing the diagnostic procedures?

A brain MRI. However, before testing could be directed by review of the brain MRI, the following work up was requested all at once, by an overambitious clinician: creatine kinase and blood smear for acanthocytes (ChAc), antigliadin antibodies (celiac disease), iron and ferritin (neuroferritinopathy), PTH and serum calcium (hypoparathyroidism), thyroid panel (TSH, Free T4; hyperthyroidism), thyroglobulin antibodies (Hashimoto thyroiditis), antiphospholipid antibody panel (antiphospholipid antibody syndrome), and ceruloplasmin. In addition, a small dose of risperidone (1 mg) was recommended for symptomatic control.

Review of the brain MRI alone could have greatly helped with narrowing the differential diagnosis by ascertaining whether there was caudate atrophy (chorea-acanthocytosis, Huntington's disease), cerebellar atrophy (spinocerebellar ataxia, celiac disease), or white matter signal abnormalities (antiphospholipid antibody syndrome).

This study showed none of the first two categories of abnormalities. Instead, it revealed confluent abnormal signal in the periventricular and deep

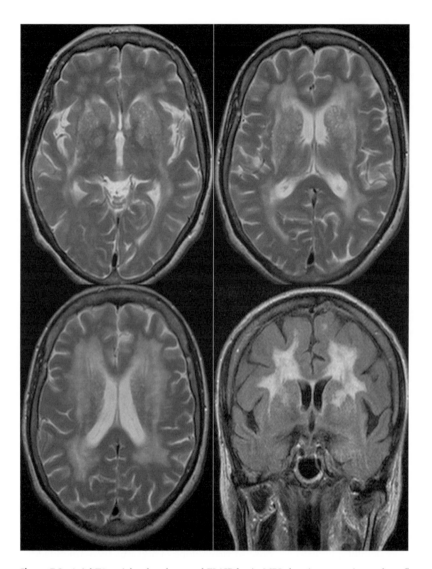

Figure 7.2. Axial T2-weighted and coronal FLAIR brain MRI showing extensive and confluent periventricular and deep white matter abnormal signal, with involvement of the basal ganglia in the form of enlargement of the perivascular spaces (Virchow-Robin spaces). These findings suggested microangiopathic brain disease as the underlying pathophysiologic mechanism associated with her chorea and tic-like disorder.

white matter regions, with widened perivascular spaces in the basal ganglia (Figure 7.2). These findings were consistent with microangiopathic brain disease and supported pursuing testing for anti-phospholipid antibodies.

But what if more than one test turns out to be "diagnostic"?

The antiphospholipid antibody panel confirmed high titers of IgG and IgM anti-cardiolipin antibodies as well as of IgG and IgM antibodies against phosphatidylserin. These abnormalities, associated with the clinical picture of chorea, epileptic events, subclinical cognitive decline, and microangiopathic brain disease, supported the diagnosis of antiphospholipid antibody syndrome. However, at the same time, abnormally high titers of antithyroglobulin ($>$ 3000 IU/mL, normal: $<$ 20) and antithyroid peroxidase antibodies (527 IU/mL, normal: $<$ 35) were reported. As her symptoms could have been explained by Hashimoto's encephalopathy, even in the absence of hypothyroidism or the subacute dementia that characterizes this disorder, the latter set of antibody abnormalities posed a dilemma hard to neglect, as the clinician was presumably suspecting this condition, and expecting to treat it, should the antibody levels be abnormal.

With a clinical picture more fully supporting antiphospholipid antibody syndrome, this patient was ultimately treated with aspirin, with stabilization of symptoms. She could have also been anticoagulated with warfarin if there had been further progression while on aspirin. The clinician was left with the lingering doubt as to whether the patient should have also been treated with steroids to address her laboratory-suggested Hashimoto's encephalopathy.

Discussion: Missing the vital piece of MRI evidence, a shot-gun approach to testing was carried out, which yielded two presumably unrelated considerations. The perils of parallel testing with simultaneous positive results are similar to those of starting two treatments at once followed by an undesirable occurrence: they become hard to interpret. Multiple or unnecessary testing may lead to false positives. For instance, a brain MRI is futile when the examination is consistent with PD – but, if requested, it may show incidental findings that could force an explanation impossible to pigeonhole into PD itself. An "unnecessary laboratory test" should be any test for which the results are not likely to truly change a diagnostic impression or the management of the patient's medical condition.[16]

Antiphospholipid antibody (or Hughes') syndrome typically presents with recurrent thrombosis, recurrent miscarriages, and neurological disease. The major pathogenic mechanism of the syndrome is vascular obstruction (both venous and arterial) due to hypercoagulability. The neurological manifestations are often the dominant feature, with headache, migraine, and cognitive dysfunction being most common while other manifestations such as dementia, epilepsy, chorea, psychiatric disease, transverse myelitis, ocular syndromes, and sensorineural hearing loss occur at a lower rate. Although chorea is the most common movement disorder associated with antiphospholipid antibody syndrome, hemidystonia, parkinsonism, tics, tremor, and myoclonus may also occur.[17] Antiaggregation therapy with aspirin or anticoagulation with warfarin can lead to significant improvement.

In this particular case, one could have complicated matters further by noting that the drugs used for this patient's treatment of rheumatoid arthritis, etanercept and leflunomide, can cause a demyelinating syndrome similar to multiple sclerosis.[18] Certainly the brain MRI may have been interpreted as suggesting such a disorder, although the lack of an increase in IgG synthesis and the absence of oligoclonal bands made this unlikely.

Diagnosis: chorea due to antiphospholipid antibody syndrome

Tip: *Do not order beyond what can be interpreted or acted upon. Always suspect antiphospholipid antibody syndrome when chorea is part of the picture in any individual with leukoencephalopathic changes on MRI.*

Case 40: Multiple negative results in tremor: perils of the exclusionary approach

Case: Six years ago, this 40-year-old woman developed abnormal movements during pregnancy that resolved completely after delivery, and were diagnosed as chorea gravidarum.

Similar movements, referred to as "post-strepto-coccal chorea," occurred 3 years later and resolved completely after 4 weeks. She had been fine until 4 days prior to presentation when she had the sudden onset of right hemibody rhythmic movements with rightward pulling of the lips, synchronous contractions of the neck, and right arm "shaking" (also reported as chorea by prior physicians). She had had about nine episodes, some accompanied by slurred speech and light-headedness, all lasting approximately 30 minutes and resolving promptly after lorazepam administration. She felt completely normal between episodes. She was no longer working as a tow truck driver.

She was examined in the midst of such an episode (Video 40). The movements recorded were acknowledged as being identical to those experienced prior to the delivery of her child and, again, after her strep throat. Tremor seemed the predominant phenotype, but the poor predictability of its frequency could have arguably been interpreted as chorea in the past. The tremor was variable and disappeared readily with distracting maneuvers. There also were intermittent platysma contractions and stuttering.

How much testing is needed before the clinical impression of psychogenic tremor is confirmed?

None. The clinical features sufficed for the diagnosis of clinically definite psychogenic tremor and no neurological investigations should be pursued. The slow tremor, which affected the lower face, neck and bilateral hands, was variable in amplitude and frequency, distractible, and entrainable and met criteria for clinically definite psychogenic tremor. The episodes reported 3 and 6 years previously as "chorea gravidarum" and "post-streptococcal chorea" may have been the same mischaracterized tremor and likely reflected conversion disorder.

Whereas the misdiagnosed chorea gravidarum is a diagnosis of exclusion, psychogenic tremor is not. Psychogenic movement disorders are diagnoses of

inclusion and meeting the criteria for each of the psychogenic phenotypes precludes the need for any additional neurological investigations. When the diagnosis is uncertain, electrophysiological tests can be very helpful in cases of tremor and myoclonus.

Discussion: A major pitfall in the assessment of these patients is when clinicians proceed with neurological investigations, even in cases meeting clinically definite criteria for psychogenic movement disorders, to "ensure that nothing is missed," even if it is to "play defensive medicine" or even to reassure patients.[19] This patient had had multiple negative investigations. The diagnosis of psychogenic tremor was considered only after extensive testing did not reveal anything of importance. This was inappropriate. Any abnormalities on testing would have represented incidental findings, irrelevant to the presentation, impossible to interpret further.

The diagnosis of psychogenic movement disorders hinges on the broad knowledge by neurologists of the variety of unusual, sometimes bizarre presentations of organic disorders. Complexity is added because psychogenic features may be seen associated with recognized movement disorders (see also Case 35 and Table 6.4); organic features, such as geste antagoniste,[20] rarely may be seen in patients with an otherwise definite psychogenic movement disorder; and *overt* psychiatric problems are often absent in these disorders.[21] Firmly diagnosing a psychogenic movement disorder and effectively communicating it to the patient prevents unnecessary testing and potentially harmful pharmacotherapy, encourages outpatient psychotherapy, and avoids "doctor shopping," which could lead to expensive and eventually unrewarding investigations, a journey to the land of permanent disability.

Diagnosis: psychogenic tremor misdiagnosed and over-investigated

Tip: *the diagnosis of psychogenic tremor should be inclusionary rather than exclusionary. No laboratory or neuroimaging investigations are indicated, except for electrophysiology to confirm selected cases of psychogenic tremor and myoclonus.*

REFERENCES

1. O'Sullivan JD, Hanagasi HA, Daniel SE, et al. Neuronal intranuclear inclusion disease and juvenile parkinsonism. *Mov Disord* 2000;**15**(5):990–995.

2. Paviour DC, Surtees RA, Lees AJ. Diagnostic considerations in juvenile parkinsonism. *Mov Disord* 2004;**19**(2):123–135.

3. Trender-Gerhard I, Sweeney MG, Schwingenschuh P, et al. Autosomal-dominant GTPCH1-deficient DRD: clinical characteristics and long-term outcome of 34 patients. *J Neurol Neurosurg Psychiatry* 2009;**80**(8):839–845.

4. Espay AJ, Paviour DC, O'Sullivan JD, et al. Juvenile levodopa-responsive Parkinsonism with early orobuccolingual dyskinesias and cognitive impairment. *Mov Disord* 2010;**25**(12):1860–1867.

5. Olsson JE, Brunk U, Lindvall B, et al. Dopa-responsive dystonia with depigmentation of the substantia nigra and formation of Lewy bodies. *J Neurol Sci* 1992;**112**(1–2):90–95.

6. Paviour DC, Revesz T, Holton JL, et al. Neuronal intranuclear inclusion disease: report on a case originally diagnosed as dopa-responsive dystonia with Lewy bodies. *Mov Disord* 2005;**20**(10):1345–1349.

7. Ito M, Matsuno K, Sakumoto Y, et al. Ataxic Guillain-Barre syndrome and acute sensory ataxic neuropathy form a continuous spectrum. *J Neurol Neurosurg Psychiatry* 2011;**82**(3):294–299.

8. Leger JM, Vaunaize J. Polyneuropathy associated with IgM monoclonal gammopathy: a review. Clinical, electrophysiological and pathological features. *Nouv Rev Fr Hematol* 1990;**32**(5):303–306.

9. Wicklund MP, Kissel JT. Paraproteinemic neuropathy. *Curr Treat Options Neurol* 2001;**3**(2):147–156.

10. Burns TM, Mauermann ML. The evaluation of polyneuropathies. *Neurology* 2011;**76**(7 Suppl 2):S6–13.

11. Klein C. Implications of genetics on the diagnosis and care of patients with Parkinson disease. *Arch Neurol* 2006;**63**(3):328–334.

12. Klein C, Schneider SA, Lang AE. Hereditary parkinsonism: Parkinson disease look-alikes – an algorithm for clinicians to "PARK" genes and beyond. *Mov Disord* 2009;**24**(14):2042–2058.

13. Valente EM, Abou-Sleiman PM, Caputo V, et al. Hereditary early-onset Parkinson's disease caused by mutations in PINK1. *Science* 2004;**304**(5674):1158–1160.

14. Williams DR, Lees AJ. How do patients with parkinsonism present? A clinicopathological study. *Intern Med J* 2009;**39**(1):7–12.

15. Riley D, Lang AE, Blair RD, et al. Frozen shoulder and other shoulder disturbances in Parkinson's disease. *J Neurol Neurosurg Psychiatry* 1989;**52**(1):63–66.

16. Griner PF, Liptzin B. Use of the laboratory in a teaching hospital. Implications for patient care, education, and hospital costs. *Ann Intern Med* 1971;**75**(2):157–163.

17. Martino D, Chew NK, Mir P, et al. Atypical movement disorders in antiphospholipid syndrome. *Mov Disord* 2006;**21**(7):944–949.

18. Al SN, Luzar MJ. Etanercept induced multiple sclerosis and transverse myelitis. *J Rheumatol* 2006;**33**(6):1202–1204.

19. Espay AJ, Goldenhar LM, Voon V, et al. Opinions and clinical practices related to diagnosing and managing patients with psychogenic movement disorders: An international survey of movement disorder society members. *Mov Disord* 2009;**24**(9):1366–1374.

20. Munhoz RP, Lang AE. Gestes antagonistes in psychogenic dystonia. *Mov Disord* 2004;**19**(3):331–332.

21. Schrag A, Lang AE. Psychogenic movement disorders. *Curr Opin Neurol* 2005;**18**(4):399–404.

8

Missing radiographic clues

Case 41: An MRI finding only seen when suspected in "PD"

Case: This 58-year-old woman was noted to "stare more" about 6 years previously. About a year later, she began to feel that her arm movements while driving were slow. A left arm tremor had developed over the last 2 years. She had occasional hypophonia and micrographia but could control the latter with effort. She noted anosmia for "as long as I can remember," endorsed frequent urination and occasionally excessive sweating, but had no constipation, skin discoloration, or postural light-headedness. Her husband reported she often shouted during her sleep and had episodes of anxiety. Pramipexole 1.5 mg/day yielded no benefits. Prior trials included amantadine (no benefit, skin mottling) and rasagiline (paradoxically, more stiffness). Her examination showed generalized hypokinesia with mild intermittent left-hand tremor, mostly evident during finger-to-nose task and on gait (Video 41a). There was decreased arm swinging on the left and mildly impaired tandem gait with preserved postural reflexes. Cognitive screen was normal (MMSE, 30; Montreal Cognitive Assessment, 29/30).

Would any testing be indicated in this case?

The case description thus far leaves little room for anything else other than PD and, regardless of the ultimate diagnostic impression, should prompt the initiation of treatment with L-dopa without any additional investigations. Comorbid anxiety and possible REM sleep behavior disorder can be held as supportive of the PD diagnosis. Obviously this case would not be highlighted here if it had not nurtured greater "visual acuity" in hindsight.

How could a brain MRI change the diagnosis and treatment?

Perhaps a brain MRI would have been requested at the first examination if this patient's imperfect tandem, the only abnormality on initial exam, had been interpreted as a "red flag" for the possible presence of an atypical parkinsonism.[1] Instead, a brain MRI was requested at her follow-up visit, 4 months later, when in addition to the welcome benefits in speech, handwriting, and walking with L-dopa, she reported the development of jaw tightness and leg wiggling, especially after each medication dose (Video 41b). This development was definitely atypical for PD, reminiscent of the L-dopa induced facial dystonia reviewed earlier in this book (see Case 13). The newly available brain MRI showed a subtle imaging abnormality, which would have been neglected had the clinician only accessed the neuroradiology report. The area of interest, often elusive to neuroradiologists not aware of the diagnostic suspicion, was a rim-like atrophy in the dorsolateral putamen, contralateral to her more affected side (Figure 8.1). This finding was critical in revising the diagnosis from PD to the parkinsonian variant of multiple system atrophy (MSA-P). This MRI finding changed the expectation

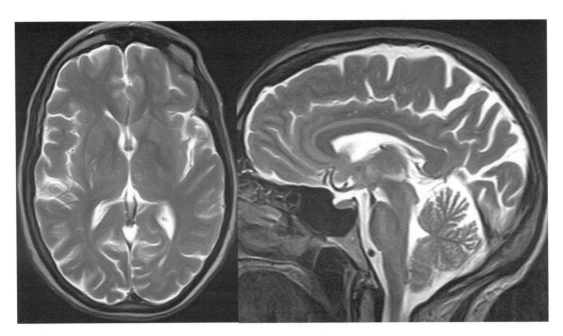

Figure 8.1. Axial and mid-sagittal T2-weighted brain MRI sequences showing subtle atrophy in the right posterolateral putamen (contralateral to the more affected side), shown as a slit-like hyperintensity, and superior cerebellar vermis. These findings are highly supportive of the clinical diagnosis of multiple system atrophy, parkinsonian variant (MSA-P). Compare with the more overt radiographic abnormalities shown in Figure 3.1.

of her future therapeutic threshold with dopaminergic drugs (higher) and the anticipation of overall survival (shorter), and helped prepare the clinician, the patient, and her family for the anticipated motor and autonomic difficulties.

Discussion: The slit-like atrophy in the posterolateral putamen may arguably be the most overlooked among the early radiologic findings in MSA-P, emerging perhaps before some of the most salient clinical features of the disorder reach full bloom. This abnormality almost never makes it onto a radiology report and can only be unearthed by a meticulous clinician, prepared to review the brain MRI independently, and mindful of the relatively small area of interest. It is possible that the early clinical clues to the diagnosis of MSA-P, namely the unusual topographic distribution of lower limb and orofacial dyskinesias, with a dystonic phenotype sometimes described as sardonic

grin,[2] lag behind the radiologic clue that ultimately clinched it. Both of these radiologic and clinical clues improve the accuracy and timeliness of the diagnosis.[3] Recognizing this combination is expected to yield a higher diagnostic accuracy than that provided by relying on the available set of diagnostic criteria.[4] PD is the most common condition with which MSA-P is confused. Other early clinical clues that should help with questioning the diagnosis of PD in patients brewing MSA-P are a tremor more prominent on action or with myoclonic features, an imperfect tandem gait, orthostatic hypotension (often not symptomatic), and greater speech involvement than one would expect in classic PD.[1;5] None of the associated historical features highlighted by this case, such as anosmia, REM sleep behavior disorder, and urination abnormalities (or other dysautonomic features for that matter), would have helped in distinguishing the two disorders.

Diagnosis: Multiple system atrophy, parkinsonian type

Tip: *the posterior putaminal atrophy will almost never be noted in neuroradiology reports and requires independent reading by the neurologist. This is a commonly missed radiographic clue, virtually pathognomonic of MSA-P. Gradient echo sequences (T2*) are often very effective in providing an early clue to the diagnosis, showing low signal in the posterior putamen, in the same region as the atrophy.*

Case 42: An MRI finding only seen when suspected in "ET"

Case: This 63-year-old man was diagnosed as having essential tremor at the age of 49 years. By age 59 years, with relatively little benefit from primidone and beta-blockers, he became dependent on his wife to perform some activities of daily living. An occasional glass of wine provided mild subjective improvement. His mother and brother had also been diagnosed as having ET. On examination, he had a right-greater-than-left, high-amplitude, low-frequency postural and action tremor that affected the upper and lower extremities (Video 42). There was no clear superimposed ataxia in the limbs, especially the legs, where it could be more reliably assessed. Handwriting was large and illegible. Tone, strength, deep tendon reflexes, and sensation were normal. Gait and stance were normal, but there was considerable instability in tandem gait.

Because of his progression, the patient underwent bilateral Vim thalamic deep brain stimulation implantation. After surgery, his limb tremor had completely resolved due to a profound microthalamotomy effect, and therefore deep brain stimulators were not turned on.

Was there any radiologic clue missed during the pre-surgical evaluation?

When this case was first examined, the significance of the brain MRI abnormalities was not known. The brain MRI showed more brain atrophy than might have been readily attributable to ET and "unusual bilateral T2 middle cerebellar hyperintensities" (Figure 8.2).[6] Immediately after surgery his balance worsened, resulting in repeated falls. His speech also became "slower." His limb tremor eventually re-emerged. The belated discovery that his grandson had fragile X syndrome, prompted testing for fragile X. His fragile X mental retardation 1 gene (*FMR1*) had 160 CGG repeats, his *FMR1* mRNA was elevated over five times the normal range, and the fragile X mental retardation 1 protein (FMRP) was reduced. These findings were diagnostic of fragile X tremor-ataxia syndrome, an ET mimic.

Discussion: Besides disabling intention tremor, this patient had impaired tandem gait, generalized brain atrophy, and, importantly, the classic bilateral T2-weighted middle cerebellar hyperintensities on brain MRI. This "MCP sign" has become the most important marker of the fragile X tremor-ataxia syndrome (FXTAS).[7] The addition of cognitive difficulties, with predominant executive deficits, completes the clinical picture. Historical features that support this diagnosis are a family history of mental retardation in boys or early menopause due to premature ovarian failure among women. This disorder is caused by elevated *FMR1* mRNA and reduced FRMP levels. Normally, *FMR1* has 6 to 40 CGG repeats. The full mutation consists of more than 200 repeats and leads to the most common genetic cause of mental retardation, fragile X syndrome (low *FMR1* mRNA).[8] The "gray zone" is considered between 41 and 54 repeats and the "premutation" carriers have 55 to 200 repeats. Thus, the same gene has the versatility of presenting at both ends of the age spectrum with two different pathogenic mechanisms: a neurodegenerative syndrome in older adults (FXTAS), caused by excess gene activity and production of a toxic RNA, and a childhood-onset disorder caused by absence of gene activity (fragile X syndrome).[9]

Incidentally, the "MCP sign" is not entirely specific for FXTAS. It has also been reported in MSA (review Figure 2.3, where there is a mild version of this sign in a case of MSA-C)[10] and acquired hepatolenticular degeneration.[11] It must be noted, however, that the

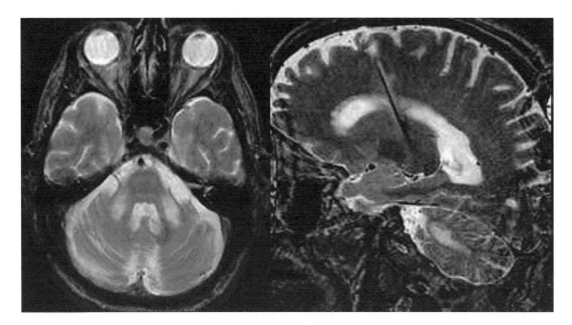

Figure 8.2. Axial and mid-sagittal T2-weighted brain MRI showing increased symmetric signal abnormality in the middle cerebellar peduncle (left) and the DBS lead and enlarged lateral ventricle resulting from generalized parenchymal atrophy. Taken with permission from Leehey et al.[6]

reported case of hepatolenticular degeneration did not show the hyperintense T1-weighted signal in the lenticular nuclei expected in patients with advanced liver disease nor was FMR1 premutation formally excluded.

Diagnosis: Fragile X tremor-ataxia syndrome (FXTAS)

Tip: *the increased signal in the middle cerebral peduncle (MCP sign) is highly suggestive of the ET-like FXTAS, particularly when progressive "essential tremor," ataxia, parkinsonism, and cognitive impairment form the clinical picture.*

Case 43: The MRI pattern of only four parkinsonisms

Case: This 55-year-old woman developed bilateral hand resting tremor and difficulty walking, with intermittent staggering while walking 5 years prior to this evaluation. L-dopa markedly improved her symptoms. However, 3 years after the onset of symptoms, she began falling, mostly backward, not predated by freezing, shuffling, festination, or a sensation of lightheadedness. Of interest, phenytoin led to a decrease in the rate of these falls but its protective effect waned over the subsequent months. She developed marked depth perception problems and often missed her target when trying to grab an object (Video 43a). She also had intermittent jerking of several body parts; she started to drop objects and had trouble feeding. Her language repertoire declined but remained grammatically correct. Her speech became softer and her face inexpressive. She stopped reading altogether. She was paranoid that her family was holding things back from her. At night, she was screaming and leaping during her sleep.

Where does the main behavioral finding localize?

Abnormalities related to depth perception localize to the dorsal stream of the visual pathway, suggesting a problem in the bilateral parieto-occipital region.

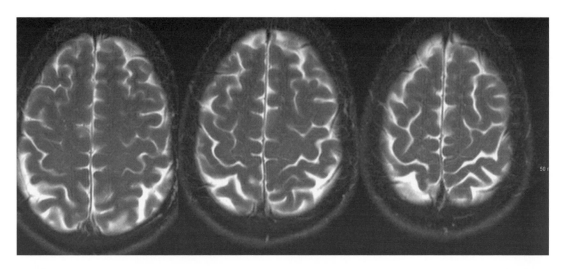

Figure 8.3. Axial T2-weighted brain MRI for the apical cuts showing narrowing of the post-central gyri and corresponding enlargement of the sulci, indicating bihemispheric parietal atrophy.

In a disorder evolving over several years, a neuro-degenerative form of posterior cortical atrophy may be localized to this area (Figure 8.3). As in Case 41, this pattern of regional atrophy is unlikely to be reported as such in a radiology report. Its ascertainment requires a clinician aware of the syndrome and its localization.

What other clinical elements should be sought?

In the setting of optic ataxia (disturbance of visually guided reaching behavior), the other clinical elements expected to be present are ocular apraxia (psychic gaze paralysis) and simultanagnosia (inability to recognize the whole from the parts). Fully developed, optic ataxia reaches its zenith when there is complete lack of visual depth perception, a situation termed astereopsis, nicely demonstrated by our patient. Together, these are the components of Balint's syndrome, a classic, if under-recognized cluster of deficits localizing to the biparieto-occipital region, a distinctive manifestation of the posterior cortical atrophy syndrome.

The relatively rapid progression of parkinsonism and dementia with prominent visuospatial impairment in the setting of Balint syndrome (optic ataxia, ocular apraxia, and simultanagnosia) suggested the presence of dementia with Lewy bodies (DLB), one of only four neurodegenerative disorders associated with the posterior cortical atrophy (PCAt) syndrome. The associated REM sleep behavior disorder is also supportive of a diagnosis of DLB.

Discussion: PCAt syndrome is both a clinical and a radiological entity. In neurodegenerative disorders, it applies to a dementing syndrome that presents with early impairment of visuospatial skills with less prominent memory loss, associated with atrophy in the parieto-occipital and posterior temporal cortices.[13] A presenile onset, illustrated in this woman, has been part of the supportive features for the proposed diagnostic criteria for PCAt.[14] Patients exhibit signs of cortical visual dysfunction either in the ventral occipitotemporal visual processing stream (the "what" pathway), such as apperceptive visual agnosia, prosopagnosia, achromatopsia, and alexia; or in the dorsal-occipitoparietal visual stream (the "where" pathway), in the form of Balint syndrome, transcortical sensory aphasia, apraxia, and some or all of the Gerstmann syndrome elements (agraphia, acalculia, finger agnosia, right-left disorientation); or in both streams (Table 8.1) (a clearer example

Table 8.1. Visual-predominant deficits resulting from the posterior cortical atrophy syndrome according to location and hemisphere predominance

	Left-predominant	Right-predominant	Bilateral
Occipital dorsal (the "where" visual pathway)	Full or partial **Balint** syndrome Contralateral **hemiachromatopsia**		Full **Balint**, poor motion perception, astereopsis
Occipital ventral (the "what" visual pathway)	**Alexia** without agraphia, upper quadrantanopsia	Apperceptive **visual agnosia**	Full-field **achromatopsia**
Occipito-temporal junction	Associative agnosia, **optic aphasia**	**Prosopagnosia and visual agnosia**	
Temporo-parietal junction	Fluent aphasia (Wernicke or transcortical sensory aphasia) Tactile object agnosia	Loss of self agency, amusia, phonagnosia	Auditory agnosia
Inferior parietal	Ideomotor apraxia, Conduction aphasia	Neglect, anosognosia, anosodiaphoria	**Balint** syndrome

All relevant visual-predominant deficits are marked in bold. Prosopagnosia is the inability to recognize familiar faces; self agency, the experience that one is the cause of one's own actions; amusia, the inability to recognize musical tones or to reproduce them. Astereopsis (lack of visual depth perception) occurs only in the setting of full Balint syndrome. Achromatopsia (black-and-white world) results from bilateral damage in the junction of the lingual with the fusiform gyrus. Anosognosia (denial of the presence of deficits) and anosodiaphoria (lack of concern for those deficits) are forms of neglect due to non-dominant inferior parietal lesions. Adapted from Espay and Biller.[12]

of Balint syndrome due to DLB is shown in Video 43b). The neurodegenerative PCAt syndrome mostly affects the dorsal visual pathways and has been the clinical domain of only four categories of disease: (1) the "visual variant" or "logopenic progressive aphasia" variant of Alzheimer's disease;[15] (2) dementia with Lewy bodies; (3) corticobasal degeneration;[16] and (4) the prion disorders Creutzfeldt-Jakob disease and fatal familial insomnia.[17] Although AD is the most common cause, with senile plaques and neurofibrillary tangles predominantly affecting visual association areas, the characteristic visuospatial problems of PCAt result from the distribution of pathology in the occipitoparietal and posterior temporal regions rather than the specific pathology itself (e.g., AD vs. DLB). Progressive prosopagnosia followed by visual object agnosia, for instance, would suggest that any of the pathologies listed above has affected the bilateral occipitotemporal

(ventral visual stream) cortices. Balint syndrome and any components of the Gerstmann syndrome would instead point to the bilateral occipitoparietal region (dorsal visual stream), again without regard for the specific pathology. Of course, parkinsonian symptoms with psychotic features in the setting of Balint syndrome would support DLB as the most likely underlying pathology.

The brain MRI of our patient showed atrophy of occipitoparietal and occipitotemporal regions and confirmed the clinical picture of PCAt.

Diagnosis: Posterior cortical atrophy presentation of dementia with Lewy bodies

Tip: *The identification of the posterior cortical atrophy syndrome yields the very short differential diagnosis of DLB, the visual variant of AD, corticobasal degeneration, and prion disorders. Balint syndrome is one of its distinctive clinical presentations.*

Case 44: Not-very-normal pressure "NPH"

Case: This 79-year-old woman developed progressive gait difficulties for 18 months prior to this evaluation. She resorted to using a walker for ambulation and often felt her knees buckle. Her balance was poor and there had been a tendency to lean to the right, though without falls. She was incontinent of urine and also had rare episodes of bowel incontinence. Her daughter reported poor insight and judgment (choked on pretzels because of not chewing them) as well as poor attention span (constantly changing television channels and not watching the movies she used to enjoy). She tended to "laugh a lot" without a clear trigger or without elation. She was referred for further evaluation for possible normal pressure hydrocephalus (NPH) based on a report of enlarged ventricles by head CT.

On exam, she showed asymmetric performance in finger tapping. She tended to lean sideways, mostly to the right. There was marked postural impairment without shortening of the stride length or widening of the base of support (Video 44a). Further examination showed pseudobulbar affect, frontal release signs (glabellar and palmomental reflexes), oculomotor dysfunction (square-wave jerks, saccadic pursuit on right gaze, and hypometric saccades) and mild dysmetria and dysdiadochokinesia on the right hand (Video 44b). The cognitive screen showed mild cognitive impairment, predominantly amnestic (MMSE = 27/30; Frontal Assessment Battery = 16/18; Montreal Cognitive Assessment = 18/30). Some of these findings suggested dysfunction of the right brainstem, prompting a review of her brain MRI (Figure 8.4).

How does the MRI evaluation change the original plan from the referring physician?

The brain MRI confirmed the focality of the neurological exam by disclosing a large extra-axial well-circumscribed isointense lesion, likely a meningioma, displacing the lower midbrain and upper pons and causing obstructive hydrocephalus.

Brainstem compression explained the right-sided predominant cerebellar deficits. The suggested work up for NPH no longer applied and a referral to one of our neurosurgery colleagues was warranted to assess for resectability of the mass and further disease-specific management.

What's the main risk for an "NPH evaluation" in this patient?

If an "NPH work up" were to have been blindly pursued without regard for the obstructive cause of her hydrocephalus, a high-volume spinal tap or a 3-day external lumbar drainage could have caused tonsillar herniation, a potentially fatal complication. Patients with a variety of NPH mimics may be harmed rather than benefited by CSF diversion procedures. Palliative ventriculoperitoneal shunt placement could only be considered in this case, if resectability of the mass were to be deemed unfeasible or too risky, only if hydrocephalus were to be considered a major contributor to the deficits.

Her presumed paramesencephalic meningioma was deemed unresectable. She died from complications of repeated aspiration pneumonia. An autopsy was not performed.

Discussion: NPH is one of the rarest but unfortunately most overdiagnosed causes of gait impairment in the elderly. The number of ventriculoperitoneal shunts placed for NPH greatly outnumbers the individuals truly affected by this disorder. Some medical centers have adopted an aggressive strategy toward suspected NPH patients by managing them with urgent large-volume taps, continuous lumbar drainage, or direct shunt placement before a careful outpatient assessment has been undertaken to determine if an alternative explanation for the gait impairment exists. True NPH is never an emergency as it should evolve slowly over years. Sustained shunt responsiveness virtually only occurs in the setting of a sequential impairment of gait first, bladder function later, and cognition last or, ideally, never when the diagnosis is made early in the process.[18]

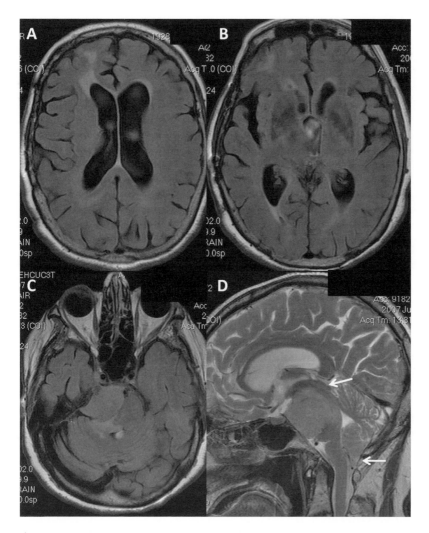

Figure 8.4. Axial FLAIR and mid-sagittal T2-weighted brain MRI showing enlarged but asymmetric lateral (A) and third ventricles (B). An isointense, relatively homogenous extraxial mass is impinging on the right pons (C) and lower midbrain (D), effacing the aqueduct (upper arrow) and displacing the tonsils downward (lower arrow).

It is important to highlight that the gait impairment of this patient was very different from that expected in individuals with true NPH (see Case 2).[19] There was no base widening, stride shortening, start hesitation, or motor blocks during turns or when approaching narrow spaces. The swaying sideways over a narrow base pointed in the direction of a hemispheric cerebellar ataxia. Admittedly,

the "syndrome of ventricular enlargement with gait apraxia" known as NPH is a difficult one to pigeon-hole, with virtually no clinicopathologic studies to support it as a defined construct and a number of associated comorbidities (hypertension, ischemic heart disease, diabetes) reported on the basis of clinical and CT-based criteria.[20] Nevertheless, NPH mimics abound and at least four patients out

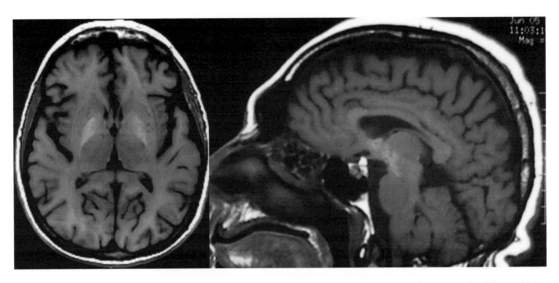

Figure 8.5. T1-weighted brain MRI demonstrating increased signal in the globus pallidus (left, axial) and midbrain (right, sagittal). Image courtesy of Dr. Leo Verhagen.

of five with suspected NPH will prove to have an alternative diagnosis after careful evaluation. Ideally such determination will be attained before and not after a shunt has been placed.

Diagnosis: Obstructive hydrocephalus due to a paramesencephalic meningioma

Tip: *Posterior fossa tumors can cause obstructive hydrocephalus, which may be misdiagnosed as NPH if examination is cursorily made and imaging abnormalities overlooked. In these patients lumbar drainage as part of a "standard NPH evaluation" is contraindicated.*

Case 45: The helpful T1-weighted MRI clue

Contributed by Dr. Leo Verhagen, Chicago, Illinois

Case: This 59-year-old developed slower gait, stooped posture, and leaning to the left while seated, followed by rest and action-induced bilateral hand tremor. Hypophonia, balance impairment, and falling were noted 1 year later. Urinary frequency, incontinence, depression, anxiety, and

obsessive compulsive behaviors became sources of disability 2 years after onset. On examination, he showed bradyphrenia, hypomimia, hypophonia, rigidity with bradykinesia and resting as well as postural tremor (Video 45). There was foot inversion and downward curling of the toes. He had an abnormal pull test. His cognitive screen was normal (MMSE = 30/30). His parkinsonism rapidly worsened. A brain MRI was obtained (Figure 8.5).

How is the T1-weighted MRI helpful?

Isolated *increased* signal in T1-weighted brain MRI helped by shortening the differential diagnosis dramatically. T1-weighted brain MRI hyperintensities do not have the long differential list that T2-weighted hyperintensities do. Only a handful of conditions can produce such a pattern and manganese is their common denominator. In this man, with elevated bilirubin, pancytopenia, and abnormal liver function tests resulting from cryptogenic liver cirrhosis, the pathogenic manganese brain accumulation represents acquired hepatolenticular degeneration. This man recovered completely after liver transplantation.

How many other conditions can this MRI appearance be associated with?

Not many. The most common is acquired hepatolenticular degeneration associated with liver failure and cirrhosis, in which blood manganese elevations correlate with the extent of pallidal hyperintensity.[21] Additional sources of manganese exposure include mining, welding, ferromanganese smelting, industrial and agricultural work, total parenteral nutrition, and ingestion of Chinese herbal pills.

Discussion: Rapidly progressive parkinsonism is always a red flag for a systemic metabolic, nutritional, toxic, or paraneoplastic process. In this setting, a brain MRI can yield the most important diagnostic clue as to the underlying etiology. Sufficient exposure to manganese will invariably result in pallidal T1-weighted brain MRI hyperintensity with *normal* T2-weighted signal, a specific biological marker of manganese accumulation.[22] A recently described form of manganese intoxication from intake of methcathinone, also causing T1-weighted hyperintensity in the pallidum, is known as "ephedronic encephalopathy." This psychostimulant is typically home-made from a combination of pseudoephedrine (Sudafed), potassium permanganate, and vinegar; melted in tap water and self administered parenterally. The large amount of potassium permanganate used as an oxidant for the chemical reaction results in the manganese-induced toxic damage of the basal ganglia. Patients thus exposed develop L-dopa-unresponsive PSP-like parkinsonism with a characteristic "cock walk."[23]

When T1- *and* T2-weighted signal are both abnormal in the pallidum, manganese toxicity is no longer a suitable explanation. In this situation, the differential diagnosis extends to include Wilson's disease, pantothenate kinase-associated neurodegeneration (neurodegeneration with brain iron accumulation 1; formerly, Hallervorden-Spatz disease), melanoma, neurofibromatosis, calcification, hyperglycemia, blood products, and fat.

Of note, iron deficiency could be an important risk factor for manganese-induced neurotoxicity as it can competitively increase manganese absorption.[24]

Hence, correcting iron deficiency is critical in the management of manganese toxicity, which may also require liver transplantation (in cases of liver cirrhosis), and avoidance of manganese supplementation in excess of $0.018\,\mu mol/kg/day$ (in cases of suspected total parenteral nutrition toxicity). Although chelation with EDTA and N-acetylcysteine have been used in cases of potassium permanganate poisoning as well as in other cases of excessive manganese exposure (e.g., mining, smelting), responses are generally poor.

Diagnosis: Acquired hepatolenticular degeneration

Tip: *Isolated T1-weighted hyperintensity in the globus pallidum represents manganese encephalopathy until proven otherwise.*

Case 46: The helpful T2* and SWI MRI clues

Contributed by Drs. Alex Lehn, Rick Boyle, Helen Brown, and George Mellick, Princess Alexandra Hospital, Brisbane, QLD, Australia

Case: This 51-year-old man had a 4-year history of dysarthria. On examination, he was noted to have excessive contraction of his frontalis muscle, oro-buccal dyskinesias and dystonic posturing of neck and left upper limb, of which he was unaware (Video 46). He had mild bradykinesia of the left upper limb. There was no dysphagia. His cognitive function was normal (MMSE = 30/30). Imaging revealed cavitations in the putamen on CT scan and marked hypointensity in the basal ganglia, motor cortex, and cerebellum on susceptibility weighted (SWI) MRI (Figure 8.6).

What should the next piece of history gathering and diagnostic testing be?

The pattern of hypointensity on SWI, which magnifies the conventional gradient echo (GRE, T2* [magnetic susceptibility gradient echo]) signal to provide maximum sensitivity to venous blood, hemorrhage, and iron storage, is most consistent with excessive iron deposition. In this setting,

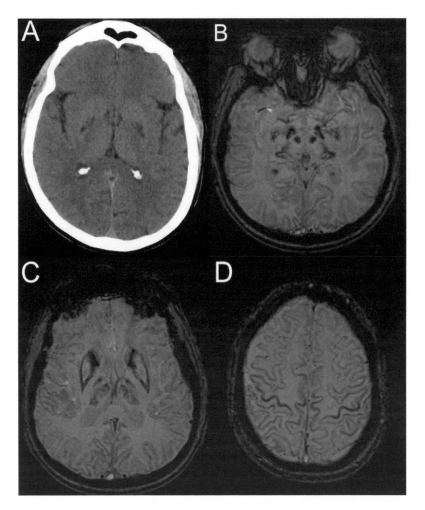

Figure 8.6. Head CT shows cavitation of the putamen (A). Axial susceptibility weighted imaging (SWI) brain MRIs show marked hypointensity in the red nuclei and substantia nigra (B), pallidum (C), and the motor strip (D).

ascertainment of family history and serum ferritin levels are the two most important history gathering and serologic diagnostic steps in determining whether neuroferritinopathy is the underlying etiology.

A strong family history was confirmed. The patient's father and three of his siblings were also affected by a similar movement disorder. Other siblings were noted to have additional clinical manifestations, including stereotypical tapping movements. Serum ferritin was 7 μg/L (normal,

30–300 μg/L). The orofacial distribution of dystonia in the setting of an autosomal dominant family history and excessive iron deposition and cavitation in the basal ganglia warranted the pursuit of genetic testing. A 460 InsA mutation in the ferritin light chain gene was confirmed. Over the subsequent 2 years, his dysarthria worsened but he remained otherwise clinically stable and cognitively intact.

Discussion: Among the neurodegeneration with brain iron accumulation (NBIA) disorders, the relatively recently recognized neuroferritinopathy (NBIA-2) may be the more frequent phenotype. Cranial dystonia and dysarthria appear to be the common clinical denominators within the NBIA disorders, which include pantothenate kinase-associated neurodegeneration (PKAN or NBIA-1; also with spasticity, generalized dystonia, and retinitis pigmentosa), aceruloplasminemia (also with diabetes and retinopathy), and infantile neuroaxonal dystrophy (INAD, also referred to as *PLA2G6*-associated neurodegeneration and PARK14).[25] The iron deposition tends to be restricted to the globus pallidus and substantia nigra in both PKAN (with an "eye of the tiger" appearance in most) and INAD, whereas it also extends into the putamen, caudate, and thalamus in neuroferritinopathy and aceruloplasminemia (with more uniform involvement and without cavitation in the latter).[26] Cavitation is a helpful neuroimaing feature in PKAN (pallidum only) and neuroferritinopathy (pallidum and putamen), as it does not occur in the other NBIA disorders, or in other neurodegenerative diseases with which there may be phenotypic similarities.[27]

Hence, there are clinical and radiologic features that overlap among the NBIA disorders. In addition to dysarthria, the development of oro-buccal dyskinesias (particularly with slow tongue movement) and stereotypical movements appear to be characteristic clinical findings in neuroferritinopathy. Remarkably, cognition remains relatively spared in these patients.

Two additional pearls from this case are worth emphasizing. First, while serum ferritin is a simple screening test when neuroferritinopathy is suspected, it can be normal even in patients with advanced disease. Even in the absence of low ferritin, in the setting of compelling clinical and neuroimaing evidence in favor of one of the NBIA disorders, genetic testing is warranted. Second, susceptibility weighted imaging has emerged as the most sensitive MRI sequence to reveal the characteristic pattern of iron deposition in the basal ganglia, motor cortex, and cerebellum. SWI is more sensitive than conventional gradient echo (GRE,

T2*-weighted) and fast-spin echo (FSE) in detecting iron, venous blood, and hemorrhage. The imaging abnormalities often develop even when the NBIA disorders are in a subclinical or mildly symptomatic early stage. Unfortunately, outcome from chelation therapy has so far been disappointing. No disease-specific treatment is currently available.

Diagnosis: Neuroferritinopathy

Tip: *The "non-routine" but widely available MRI sequence SWI is most sensitive in ascertaining iron deposition in the basal ganglia, helping steer the diagnosis toward neuroferritinopathy or one of the other neurodegeneration with brain iron accumulation disorders.*

REFERENCES

1. Abdo WF, Borm GF, Munneke M, et al. Ten steps to identify atypical parkinsonism. *J Neurol Neurosurg Psychiatry* 2006;**77**(12):1367–1369.

2. Wenning GK, Geser F, Poewe W. The 'risus sardonicus' of multiple system atrophy. *Mov Disord* 2003; **18**(10):1211.

3. Osaki Y, Wenning GK, Daniel SE, et al. Do published criteria improve clinical diagnostic accuracy in multiple system atrophy? *Neurology* 2002;**59**(10): 1486–1491.

4. Hughes AJ, Daniel SE, Ben-Shlomo Y, et al. The accuracy of diagnosis of parkinsonian syndromes in a specialist movement disorder service. *Brain* 2002;**125**(Pt 4): 861–870.

5. Litvan I, Goetz CG, Jankovic J, et al. What is the accuracy of the clinical diagnosis of multiple system atrophy? A clinicopathologic study. *Arch Neurol* 1997;**54**(8):937–944.

6. Leehey MA, Munhoz RP, Lang AE, et al. The fragile X premutation presenting as essential tremor. *Arch Neurol* 2003;**60**(1):117–121.

7. Cohen S, Masyn K, Adams J, et al. Molecular and imaging correlates of the fragile X-associated tremor/ataxia syndrome. *Neurology* 2006;**67**(8):1426–1431.

8. Chonchaiya W, Schneider A, Hagerman RJ. Fragile X: a family of disorders. *Adv Pediatr* 2009;**56**:165–186.

9. Amiri K, Hagerman RJ, Hagerman PJ. Fragile X-associated tremor/ataxia syndrome: an aging face of the fragile X gene. *Arch Neurol* 2008;**65**(1):19–25.

10. Storey E, Billimoria P. Increased T2 signal in the middle cerebellar peduncles on MRI is not specific for fragile X premutation syndrome. *J Clin Neurosci* 2005;**12**(1):42–43.

11. Lee J, Lacomis D, Comu S, et al. Acquired hepatocerebral degeneration: MR and pathologic findings. *AJNR Am J Neuroradiol* 1998;**19**(3):485–487.

12. Espay AJ, Biller J. *Concise Neurology.* Philadelphia, PA: Lippincott Williams & Wilkins, division of Wolters Kluwer Health, Inc., 2011.

13. Kirshner HS, Lavin PJ. Posterior cortical atrophy: a brief review. *Curr Neurol Neurosci Rep* 2006;**6**(6):477–480.

14. Tang-Wai DF, Graff-Radford NR, Boeve BF, et al. Clinical, genetic, and neuropathologic characteristics of posterior cortical atrophy. *Neurology* 2004;**63**(7):1168–1174.

15. Ross SJ, Graham N, Stuart-Green L, et al. Progressive biparietal atrophy: an atypical presentation of Alzheimer's disease. *J Neurol Neurosurg Psychiatry* 1996;**61**(4):388–395.

16. Wadia PM, Lang AE. The many faces of corticobasal degeneration. *Parkinsonism Relat Disord* 2007;**13** Suppl 3:S336–S340.

17. Renner JA, Burns JM, Hou CE, et al. Progressive posterior cortical dysfunction: a clinicopathologic series. *Neurology* 2004;**63**(7):1175–1180.

18. Black PM. Idiopathic normal-pressure hydrocephalus: results of shunting in 62 patients. *J Neurosurg* 1980;**52** (3):371–377.

19. Giladi N, Kao R, Fahn S. Freezing phenomenon in patients with parkinsonian syndromes. *Mov Disord* 1997;**12**(3):302–305.

20. Casmiro M, D'Alessandro R, Cacciatore FM, et al. Risk factors for the syndrome of ventricular enlargement with gait apraxia (idiopathic normal pressure hydrocephalus): a case-control study. *J Neurol Neurosurg Psychiatry* 1989;**52**(7):847–852.

21. Hauser RA, Zesiewicz TA, Martinez C, et al. Blood manganese correlates with brain magnetic resonance imaging changes in patients with liver disease. *Can J Neurol Sci* 1996;**23**(2):95–98.

22. Josephs KA, Ahlskog JE, Klos KJ, et al. Neurologic manifestations in welders with pallidal MRI T1 hyperintensity. *Neurology* 2005;**64**(12):2033–2039.

23. Stepens A, Logina I, Liguts V, et al. A Parkinsonian syndrome in methcathinone users and the role of manganese. *N Engl J Med* 2008;**358**(10):1009–1017.

24. Herrero HE, Valentini MC, Discalzi G. T1-weighted hyperintensity in basal ganglia at brain magnetic resonance imaging: are different pathologies sharing a common mechanism? *Neurotoxicology* 2002;**23**(6):669–674.

25. McNeill A, Chinnery PF. Neurodegeneration with brain iron accumulation. *Handb Clin Neurol* 2011;**100**:161–172.

26. McNeill A, Birchall D, Hayflick SJ, et al. T2* and FSE MRI distinguishes four subtypes of neurodegeneration with brain iron accumulation. *Neurology* 2008;**70**(18):1614–1619.

27. Schneider SA, Walker RH, Bhatia KP. The Huntington's disease-like syndromes: what to consider in patients with a negative Huntington's disease gene test. *Nat Clin Pract Neurol* 2007;**3**(9):517–525.

9

Management misadventures

Case 47: "Rapidly progressing" PD

Case: This 74-year-old man first developed a resting tremor in the right index finger 16 years ago, at the age of 58 years. He started experiencing some shuffling about 6 years later, and began to use a cane to help with stability 2 years ago. He was still able to walk 3 miles per day until about 6 weeks prior to this evaluation, when he rapidly declined, and over days he became unable to walk at all, being virtually confined to a wheelchair. The tremor worsened in a jerky fashion and he started to fall for the first time. He also developed red discoloration of the legs and difficulty with thinking and memorizing. His speech softened and he had a few choking episodes.

He was treated with pramipexole 1.5 mg q.i.d. (6 mg/day), carbidopa/L-dopa 150/entacapone (CLE [Stalevo] 150), 1 tablet q.i.d., sustained release carbidopa/L-dopa (sinemet CR 25/100), 0.5 tablets q.i.d., amantadine 100 mg t.i.d., and clonazepam 1 mg at bedtime.

On examination, he showed resting and postural myoclonic movements in the hands and neck, intermittent and jerky large-amplitude right-hand tremor, and marked postural and gait impairments. He could barely take a few steps beyond his wheelchair. He also had livedo reticularis in the thighs (Video 47a). He qualified as mildly demented according to the basic cognitive screen (MMSE = 21/30).

What are the clues to this man's severe disability?

The rapidity of his deterioration with a defined, rather abrupt, downturn makes one highly suspicious of factors extrinsic to PD, such as infections, metabolic derangements, or drugs. The latter category became immediately suspect when considering that his wheelchair-bound status was reached within 2 months from the initiation of treatment with amantadine 300 mg/day. It is highly probable that amantadine accounted for the development of myoclonus, livedo reticularis, and cognitive impairment, whereas an insufficient dose of L-dopa (only 600 mg/day of the immediate release formulation) may have been responsible for the worsening postural impairment and freezing. The dose of pramipexole (6 mg/day) was excessive for most patients and this may have contributed to his cognitive impairment and leg edema.

What to do next?

In prioritized sequence, one should first discontinue amantadine, the most likely cause of his greatest disability, reduce the dose of pramipexole to 4.5 mg/day (within the recommended therapeutic range), and increase dopaminergic stimulation by increasing the dose of CLE from 150 to 200 per dose.

After these changes were enacted, despite the emergence of non-troublesome levodopa-induced dyskinesias, he resumed independent

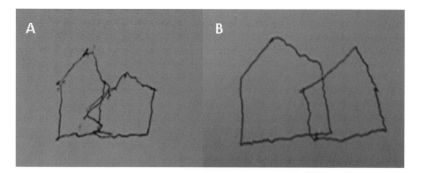

Figure 9.1. Intercepting pentagon task performance at the initial visit (A) and 2 months after the discontinuation of amantadine (B). Note the reduction in the jerkiness and the better reproduction of the requested task.

ambulation and reported a resolution of falls, improvement in cognition, disappearance of leg discoloration, and strengthening of his speech. His exam showed restoration of gait and substantially reduced tremor (Video 47b). Postural myoclonus was markedly reduced (Figure 9.1). His motor function improved 200%, as measured by the motor subscale of the UPDRS (from 64 to 22/ 108, lower is better) and his subjective cognitive benefits were matched by gains in the MMSE (from 21 to 25/30). His livedo reticularis was no longer apparent.

Discussion: This case is highly instructive for several reasons. First, it demonstrates the capacity of the standard PD pharmacotherapy to harm, when inappropriately used. The treatment was based on a supra-therapeutic (toxic) dose of a dopamine agonist and a subtherapeutic dose of L-dopa, a strategy that can readily backfire in anyone over the age of 65 years. Further, it depended on the CR formulation of L-dopa, which is notoriously unreliable from a pharmacokinetic perspective (probably more so when half-tablet doses are used). The Practice Parameter on the treatment of motor fluctuations and dyskinesia, issued by the Quality Standards Subcommittee of the American Academy of Neurology, in fact suggested that sinemet CR "may be disregarded to reduce off time" (Level C recommendation) due to its unpredictable absorption and dose response.[1]

Importantly, in addition to the rapid, uncharacteristic decline of function in a non-demented, previously well-controlled PD patient, the predominantly myoclonic phenotype should have been interpreted as a red flag. Amantadine was the most likely culprit given the combination of myoclonus (see also Case 18), cognitive impairment, and livedo reticularis.[2] Amantadine is best reserved for cases of dyskinesia not sufficiently improved with manipulations in the dosage of dopaminergic therapies.[3] It can provide additional antiparkinsonian benefit but should be used cautiously in view of its side effect profile, in particular, cognitive impairment with or without hallucinations, though these also develop with many antiparkinson medications including anticholinergics and dopaminergic drugs.[4]

In addition to mistreatment, undertreatment with subtherapeutic doses of dopaminergic medications may be the most common reason for "treatment-refractory" PD. There is a common misperception among patients, not aggressively contested by physicians, that doing with less medication now will be better for tomorrow, particularly as it applies to the risk of levodopa-induced dyskinesias or a theoretical finite duration of L-dopa effect. In fact, short-changing patients' dopaminergic replacement decreases their quality of life and may be deleterious in the long term.[5] The risk of dyskinesias should not be held as sufficient argument to maintain treatment at a subtherapeutic level.

Diagnosis: Parkinson's disease, mismanaged

Tip: *Dopamine agonists and amantadine must be used with extreme caution in PD patients older than 65 years given the increasingly poor risk/benefit ratio with age. Undertreatment is a very common cause of "poorly responsive" PD.*

Case 48: From orofacial dyskinesias to worse

Case: Constant movements of her jaws, lips, and tongue were first brought to the attention of this 63-year-old woman about 2 years prior to presentation. She had been on treatment with aripiprazole for several years to address severe depression and anxiety, which had kept her from working as a nurse. Tardive dyskinesia was suspected. She was switched to quetiapine and benztropine but neither her depression nor her abnormal movements were controlled. Over the subsequent months, she started to notice short-term memory impairment and episodes of crying; she became less interested in cooking and carrying out domestic chores. She also developed an action tremor, most noticeable when using silverware. She would chew food more than before, the tongue tended to stick out (though not necessarily when chewing), her lips became chapped, and she began to fall.

On exam, the orolingual movements were not readily apparent to her. Her speech was not affected and there was no tongue protrusion impersistence (Video 48a). There was mild dystonic posturing in the fingers, action-induced tremor, rigidity in the arms and neck, and fatiguing of rapid alternating movements, suggesting mild parkinsonism. Postural reflexes were impaired.

What was the main pitfall in her management?

Although her diagnosis was correctly suspected as representing classic tardive dyskinesia, her management was based on adding an anticholinergic drug to her regimen. This approach may work well in the tardive dystonia form of tardive dyskinesia, but is often counterproductive in classic (or buccolinguomasticatory) tardive dyskinesia, causing worsening of the movements and overall decompensation. This experience emphasizes the importance of distinguishing the tardive syndromes by phenotype, as the treatment strategy differs between them.

What to do next?

Benztropine and quetiapine were sequentially removed and replaced with paroxetine to address her depression and anxiety. Three months later, the movements of her jaws, lips, and tongue had virtually disappeared. Her lips were no longer chapped as before. Her balance had also improved and her parkinsonism improved by 50% (as measured by the motor subscale of the UPDRS). Her cognitive function normalized (MMSE changed from 19/30 to 28/30). At the 1 year follow-up, she remained much improved (Video 48b). Paroxetine 10 mg was completely controlling her depression.

Discussion: Although tardive syndromes often coexist, classic or buccolinguomasticatory tardive dyskinesia rarely presents concurrently with one of its subcategories, tardive dystonia, from which it can be distinguished clinically. Tardive dystonia tends to affect the lower face, often impairs speech, and may be associated with the classic combination of retrocollis, paroxysmal arching backwards of the trunk, internal rotation of the arms, extension at the elbows, and flexion at the wrists (Video 48c).[6] Classic tardive dyskinesia presents largely as orofacial chorea and rarely affects speech or extends beyond the orofacial region. It is characterized by repetitive tongue twisting and protrusion, and purposeless puckering, lip smacking, pursing, and chewing. These clinical distinctions suggest differences in pathophysiology and, correspondingly, response to treatment between these two tardive syndromes (Table 9.1). In particular, as illustrated by this case, while anticholinergic agents

Table 9.1. Clinical and management differences between classic tardive dyskinesia and the subcategory of tardive dystonia

Feature	Classic tardive dyskinesia	Tardive dystonia
Nature	Resulting from cumulative (intermittent) exposure to neuroleptics	Most frequent form of symptomatic dystonia, presumed idiosyncratic
Age and gender	Older females	Young males
Topographic extension	Oro-bucco-lingual region predominates	Segmental extension common
Speech	Usually unaffected	Typically affected
Preferred treatment	No convincingly good treatment.* Dopaminergic and anticholinergic agents may increase its severity	Dopamine depletors (reserpine, tetrabenazine) and anticholinergics

* Tetrabenazine may be effective but side effects (e.g., drug-induced parkinsonism) commonly limit its efficacy.

are helpful in tardive dystonia, these drugs, as well as dopamine agonists, tend to exacerbate tardive dyskinesia.[7] Hence, the recognition of these disorders, and their differences, should help with the appropriate selection of pharmacotherapy. The desirable withdrawal of the offending agent, which should never be abrupt, may in fact cause, at least initially, symptomatic worsening. When this withdrawal is not feasible, the atypical antipsychotic risperidone has been advocated to improve tardive dyskinesia.[8] Another option is to switch to clozapine, which may have an active pharmacologic anti-tardive dyskinesia effect.[9] When direct anti-dyskinetic pharmacotherapy becomes necessary in patients with very severe, disabling forms of tardive dyskinesia, the dopamine depleting drug tetrabenazine (or, in sequence, reserpine or alpha-methyl-paratyrosine)

may be considered as a first-line treatment but depression, akathisia, and parkinsonism frequently occur. Second-line agents reported include clonazepam, beta-blockers, amantadine, and levetiracetam.[10]

Finally, although incidence data are lacking, the atypical antipsychotics aripiprazole (as in this case), olanzapine, risperidone, and ziprasidone, possibly safer than their typical counterparts, have all been associated with the development of tardive dyskinesia.[11]

Diagnosis: Tardive dyskinesia, worsened by treatment with an anticholinergic

Tip: *Anticholinergic agents tend to increase the severity of tardive dyskinesia, a key difference with tardive dystonia, and one of the reasons to distinguish these complications of neuroleptic drugs.*

Case 49: Shunt-unresponsive "NPH"

Case: This 72-year-old man a with history of hyperlipidemia, hypertension, hypercholesterolemia, and left frontal lobe stroke developed stuttering of gait 2 years prior to his evaluation. His balance progressively worsened, especially when turning, with a tendency to lean to the right. Within 2 years, he was falling at least three times weekly without lightheadedness or any warning signs. He was using a wheelchair for transportation purposes outside his home but often ambulated without assistance at home. He also complained of occasional choking when swallowing liquids with his head turned back. He had experienced urinary incontinence for about 3 years and had occasional bowel incontinence. His brain MRI was interpreted as demonstrating hydrocephalus disproportionate to the degree of parenchymal atrophy (Figure 9.2). His exam confirmed truncal ataxia and mild dementia (MMSE = 24; Montreal Cognitive Assessment = 13/30) and these findings were argued to suggest normal pressure hydrocephalus (Video 49a). Impairment of upgaze with absent vertical optokinetic responses was recognized and acknowledged as atypical for

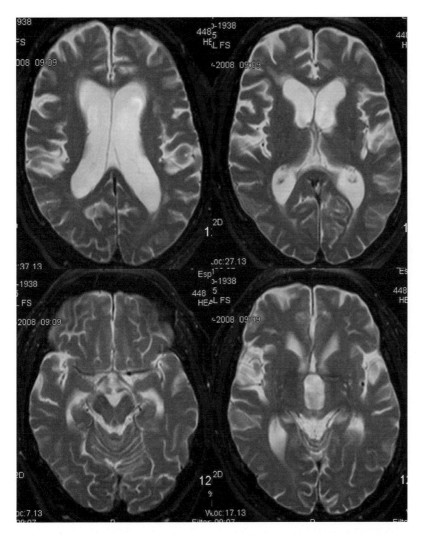

Figure 9.2. Axial T2-weighted brain MRI demonstrating hydrocephalus, interpreted as disproportionate to the degree of surrounding atrophy. Early red flags, which were missing from the initial assessment of this study, were atrophy of the tegmental midbrain with lack of a true hydrocephalic convexity at the temporal horns of the lateral ventricles (left lower image) and a disproportionately prominent ex-vacuo enlargement of the third ventricle (right lower image).

NPH but the overall "burden of evidence" was felt to favor this disorder.

It was decided to proceed with an admission to the hospital for 3 days of external lumbar drainage (ELD) with before-and-after neuropsychological evaluations and gait analyses in order to determine his suitability for ventriculoperitoneal shunt (VPS) placement.

What is the major pitfall regarding this decision?

The decision to consider VPS placement was based on flawed assumptions. The clinical history and the MRI findings poked a number of holes in the NPH diagnosis. From a clinical perspective, falls and oculomotor impairment within 2 years from the

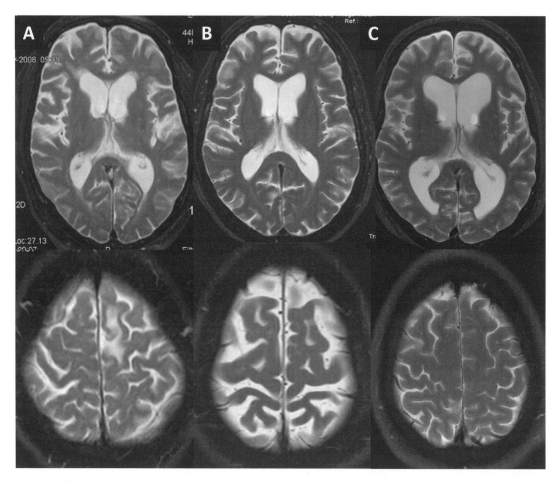

Figure 9.3. Axial T2-weighted brain MRI at the level of the lateral ventricles (upper row) and corresponding apical cuts (lower row) for this case of shunt-unresponsive "NPH" (A), a patient with mild dementia of Alzheimer's type (B) and and a patient with shunt-responsive NPH (C). The larger ventricular size of C is associated with a pattern of packed gyri in the apical cuts, unlike that in A and B. Predominant biparietal atrophy is appreciated in B compared with A and C (old left frontal stroke is noted in A). A and B patients were inappropriately considered as potential "NPH candidates." Compare with Figure 1.3.

onset of symptoms strongly argued against NPH. Choking on swallowing liquids should have raised important concerns about the proposed diagnosis. From an imaging standpoint, the parenchymal atrophy should have elicited apprehension. Inspection of the apical cuts demonstrated absence of the packed gyri with minimal sulcation that would have supported NPH (Figure 9.3, compare with Figure 1.3). Instead, the sulci widening

approached that seen in a neurodegenerative disorder (e.g., AD, Figure 9.3B) rather than NPH (Figure 9.3C). Of greater etiologic significance than the generalized brain atrophy, the disproportionate enlargement of the third ventricle compared with the lateral ventricles (Figure 9.2, right lower corner) should have alerted the clinician to the presence of the more specific mesencephalic atrophy. Indeed, review of the mid-sagittal brain MRI revealed atrophy

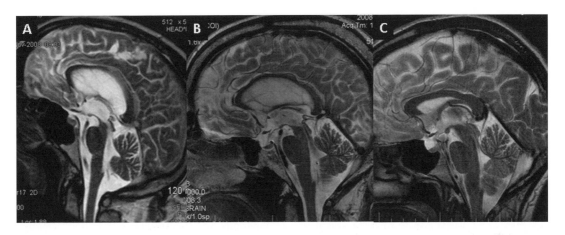

Figure 9.4. Mid-sagittal T2-weighted brain MRI in this shunt-unresponsive case (A), a patient with shunt-responsive NPH (B), and an age-matched normal adult (C). Notice the atrophy of the brainstem, particularly midbrain (giving it a "hummingbird" appearance), and associated ex-vacuo enlargement of the aqueduct in A compared with B and C, in part from thinning of the superior cerebellar peduncle (not shown).

of the midbrain, cerebellar vermis, and superior cerebellar peduncle (Figure 9.4).

The 3-day ELD procedure led to some improvement in stride length (~20%) and modestly (<10%) in gait velocity. However, there was moderate objective motor deterioration (UPDRS worsened 5 points) and no cognitive benefits (he remained in a similarly impaired range for most cognitive endpoints). Given subjective overall benefits reported by the family in balance, mood, and urinary continence, a decision was eventually made to proceed with VPS placement.

Six months after VPS placement, he had shown less urinary incontinence but his mood had become irritable. His gait had a wider base and he required help with ambulation at all times. He had fallen several times, all backwards. He was holding the silverware in an incorrect manner for the first time. He had trouble finding words. Exam demonstrated greater impairment of upgaze and slower vertical saccades, with appearance of the "round the houses" sign, the accomplishment of impaired vertical saccades by moving the eyes in a lateral arc (i.e., lateropulsion) (Video 49b). This bedside sign has been proposed as helpful in the early diagnosis of PSP, when the supranuclear vertical gaze palsy is

not fully developed.[12] He went on to develop frontal release signs with disinhibition and worsening of executive dysfunction, facial dystonia, and more severe postural impairment complicated by backward falls. He became wheelchair-bound within 3 years of symptom onset and died a year later from complications of aspiration pneumonia. Brain autopsy confirmed the final clinical diagnosis of PSP.

Discussion: Communicating hydrocephalus in the elderly is overdiagnosed as NPH. Only a careful history and neurologic examination and review of imaging data can reveal the correct diagnosis before shunt-unresponsiveness helps define it by exclusion. This case illustrates an NPH mimic that should have been apparent at the initial evaluation had the history of early falls and exam findings of oculomotor impairment been given proper diagnostic weight. VPS placement created a brief, mostly subjective improvement followed by a more rapid deterioration. A clearer picture of PSP ultimately emerged.

PSP is among the neurodegenerative disorders that may be associated with hydrocephalus potentially misinterpreted as representing NPH. Interestingly, temporary improvements in gait and bladder control have been documented in PSP patients with radiologic hydrocephalus subjected to shunting procedures.[13] In these patients, upward gaze was most restricted early on, with relative preservation of downward and horizontal saccades. Also, early shunt responsiveness was reported in three out of five patients with possible NPH and parkinsonism who evolved into a picture of PSP (one pathology proven).[14] Mass effects of hydrocephalus or changes secondary to ventriculomegaly impacting on cortico-striato-pallido-thalamo-cortical circuit have been proposed as potentially inducing parkinsonism in hydrocephalus.[14] Alternatively, a more aggressive neurodegenerative disorder (such as in this case, with a 4-year disease course) could plausibly generate hydrocephalus by an ex-vacuo mechanism. It has been suggested that PSP, AD, and vascular dementia result in an alteration in the compliance of cerebral tissue, especially in the periventricular region. The relatively poor long-term response rates of shunting for "NPH" is probably due to this association between a "hydrodynamic" component of hydrocephalus in some patients with progressive neurodegenerative diseases. The possibility that hydrocephalus can accompany these disorders should greatly emphasize clinical scrutiny of history, exam, and imaging to unravel their true nature and minimize the temptation to offer shunting to these patients.[15]

Diagnosis: Progressive supranuclear palsy, with shunt-unresponsive hydrocephalus

Tip: *Dementia preceding gait and urinary dysfunction, rather than following these deficits, is suggestive of an NPH mimic, most likely a neurodegenerative dementia or dementia-parkinsonism disorder. Falls and oculomotor impairment are never part of the spectrum of true NPH.*

Case 50: Replacing one deficit with another

Case: This 54-year-old man complained of progressive difficulties with speech and swallowing. He had noted that using a tooth pick minimized the jaw

movements. Increased involuntary blinking also developed. He gradually became socially isolated and lost interest in social activities. He had not had exposure to neuroleptics. Exam showed isolated dystonic contractions of several cranial muscles associated with intermittent tongue protrusion (Video 50a). Treatment with tetrabenazine, increased to a dose of 75 mg daily, provided clear but insufficient benefits (Video 50b). The dose was increased in order to optimize his response but, as he reached a dose of 125 mg/day, residual dystonia was replaced with parkinsonian features of masked facies, tongue tremor, and slowed gait (Video 50c). Tapering of tetrabenazine caused rebound worsening of the craniofacial dystonia (Video 50d).

What were the main pitfalls in the management of this patient?

Twofold: first, botulinum toxin chemodenervation should have been offered as first line of treatment given its efficacy and the favorable side effect profile in focal dystonias, compared to available oral medications (anticholinergics, tetrabenazine, baclofen, and benzodiazepines, among others). Second, although the development of parkinsonism with tetrabenazine may not have been preventable, the rebound worsening was prompted by a rapid tapering process. Re-exposing patients to a lower dose of tetrabenazine once withdrawal worsening has occurred may not provide a similar magnitude of benefit.

Discussion: The topographical involvement of cranial and cervical muscles in the form of blepharospasm, oromandibular, and neck dystonia defines segmental craniocervical dystonia. A common etiology is chronic exposure to neuroleptics,[16] which if it had been applicable to this patient would have warranted discontinuation of the offending drug as the first line of treatment. As in this idiopathic form of craniofacial dystonia, the tardive variant may also affect speech and chewing and cause difficulty with jaw opening and closing (see Video 48c). Although modest benefit can be achieved with some of the oral agents, including anticholinergics, baclofen, and benzodiazepines, the best opportunity for improvement may come from the use of tetrabenazine but, as this case illustrated, the therapeutic threshold may be dangerously close to the toxic one. These patients are currently best managed with chemodenervation using any of the available botulinum toxins.[17] Only in refractory cases pallidal deep brain stimulation may be offered.[18]

Incidentally, the descriptive labels "cranial dystonia" and "segmental craniocervical dystonia" have been proposed to replace the eponymic term "Meige sydrome." This nomenclature eliminates confusion by eliminating the implied "facial" distribution of this focal dystonia, since the masticatory muscles neither arise in nor attach to the face but rather to the cranium and/or mandible.[19]

Diagnosis: segmental cranial dystonia

Tip: *Tetrabenazine increases the risk of parkinsonism. A dose reduction or elimination when used to treat dystonia may induce rebound worsening. Local chemodenervation is the preferred treatment for segmental dystonias.*

Case 51: "This is not my husband"

Case: This 51-year-old man had classical PD symptoms for about 10 years, which started with left-hand tremor and left foot dragging when walking. He had shown excellent benefits with a combination of L-dopa (IR and CR formulations combined), entacapone, ropinirole, selegiline, and amantadine, although he was experiencing wearing off in the form of painful foot dystonia and diphasic dyskinesias. His wife reported that, for about the last 3 years, he ate and drank whatever was placed in front of him, which was uncharacteristic. She also noted that he had increasing interest in pornography, and he started to purchase pornographic DVDs, buy rubber penis devices from sex shops, and was taking pictures of himself using sexual objects. She perceived that his decision making was impaired and, "unlike the

husband I knew, he is doing things without regards for personal safety."

What is the iatrogenic problem and how to sort it out?

This man developed impulse control disorders (ICDs), the failure to resist an impulse to perform an activity that is pleasurable but harmful to the person and/or to others. In him, ICDs manifested as compulsive eating and pornography seeking, traits that are unlike the typical risk aversive personality of PD. With as many antiparkinsonian treatments as he was on, any of the dopaminergic drugs could in isolation (or perhaps, in combination) be considered as causative of his behavioral complication. As dopamine agonists are the most commonly reported offending agents, a tapering with discontinuation of ropinirole was recommended as the next most appropriate step.

Within a week after the elimination of ropinirole, there was improvement of pornography seeking and hypersexuality but some residual activity in these behaviors remained. The patient addressed longer off periods by adding two doses of CR L-dopa. Over the next few months, although he was no longer engaged in pornography, he was shoplifting anything with phallic significance, which he used for self stimulation. He did not seem to immediately recognize the perils of his behavior but would eventually acknowledge them as wrong. His motor function had been otherwise relatively stable with only mild diphasic dyskinesias and wearing off in the evening.

Why was there a short honeymoon in therapeutic response?

It is unclear; however, any dopaminergic agents can elicit ICDs as a complication. It is possible that the replacement of ropinirole with doses of CR L-dopa presumably equally effective for motor dysfunction may not have sufficiently altered the cerebral dysfunction causing the ICDs. Alternatively, the erratic absorption of the CR formulation of L-dopa may have preserved the abnormal pharmacodynamic complication. To ease interpretation of the drug effects in this patient and complying with the AAN's recommendation that daytime use of CR L-dopa should be avoided in complex fluctuators,[1] it would be appropriate to simplify the drug regimen by converting CR L-dopa entirely to the IR formulation.

After this change, in addition to improving his wearing off periods, his behaviors of self stimulation markedly decreased and he no longer engaged in pornography. A neuropsychological evaluation demonstrated mild cognitive impairment (Mattis DRS-2 = 125 [borderline]; MoCA = 22/30) with predominant difficulty on executive tasks but no depression or personality disorders.

Discussion: ICDs have emerged as a medico-legal pitfall in the treatment of PD. Expressed in the form of problematic or pathological gambling, compulsive sexual behavior, compulsive buying, and binge-eating disorder, ICDs complicate treatment in nearly 15% of PD patients, about three times more in patients with than without a dopamine agonist.[20] Risk factors include younger age, levodopa use, cigarette smoking, alcohol abuse, high novelty-seeking personality traits, and a family history of gambling problems. Amantadine has also been associated with the development of ICDs.[21] ICDs need to be distinguished from dopamine dysregulation syndrome (DDS), largely an addictive behavior triggered by short-acting drugs such as L-dopa and apomorphine, whereby patients seek a hypomanic state by increasing the dosage or frequency of L-dopa or apomorphine, often also causing severe dyskinesias.[22]

The highly specific affinity for brain D_3 receptors, known to be localized to the mesolimbic system, may be at the root of the pathologic behaviors unleashed by dopamine agonists to an extent greater than other dopaminergic drugs.[23] It is important to counsel patients on this potential risk and monitor for its development regularly, before any of the emerging ICDs undermine the individual's family, social, or occupational environment. Reliance on the lowest

effective doses of dopamine agonists may lower the risk of developing ICDs. However, these behaviours can occur with low doses, as used to treat RLS.

Diagnosis: Impulse control disorder complicating PD treatment

Tip: *Warn patients and spouses about the potential for ICDs, and monitor for their development, especially when using dopamine agonists in young PD patients, particularly if there is a history of novelty-seeking personality traits and gambling problems.*

Case 52: "This is *definitely* not my husband"

Case: This 58-year-old man noted forgetfulness and "scatter mindedness" 3 years before the development of right-hand tremor, which prompted the diagnosis of PD. For many years prior, he was known to shout and leap out of bed during his sleep. Shortly after diagnosis, he was noted to veer off to the sides when walking and have episodes of sudden-onset disorientation and postural lightheadedness. Falls, most of them backward, began to occur by the fourth year of illness, when he was also noted to have problems with "judging distances". Treatment with pramipexole led to excessive daytime sedation and compulsive shopping, and was discontinued. L-dopa improved the tremor but caused visual hallucinations, multiple episodes of agitation, paranoia, and tactile hallucinations, whereby he wanted to "rip his face off." Olanzapine was introduced to address these problems. His wife reported him to be much worse and sent us a video of a nocturnal event for our review (Video 52).

What was the treatment misadventure and how to redress it?

Initiation of olanzapine (or, for that matter, most other atypical antipsychotics) was bound to worsen a PD-like disorder with early cognitive impairment and fluctuations as well as L-dopa-induced psychosis. Although a misadventure of sorts, this "neuroleptic sensitivity" helped to further confirm the suspicion (assuming there was one) that dementia with Lewy bodies (DLB) was this patient's underlying disorder. Though the clues to the appropriate diagnosis were apparent before treatment with olanzapine, this apparently paradoxical response to an atypical neuroleptic further clarified the diagnosis. In addition to his parkinsonism and psychosis, examination of this patient within 5 years of disease onset revealed dementia with predominant visuospatial and executive impairment (MMSE = 21/30; Montreal Cognitive Assessment = 19/30) and mild non-transitive ideomotor apraxia. His long-standing dream enactment behaviors suggested comorbid REM sleep behavior disorder (RBD) and supported the likelihood of a synucleinopathy being the underlying pathology. DLB in particular is often heralded by RBD years or decades before, and by visuospatial disorientation at or shortly after, the onset of motor deficits.[24]

Replacing olanzapine with quetiapine or, ideally, clozapine is recommended to enhance control of psychosis without the motor and even behavioral worsening induced more commonly by other antipsychotics. In this patient, treatment with clozapine decreased hallucinations but dose increases were progressively needed to compensate for more prominent psychotic bouts. Clonazepam markedly abated his RBD-associated dream enactment behaviors. Toward his death, about 8 years from symptom onset, and despite levodopa dose adjustments and increases in clozapine, he experienced increasing akathisia and psychotic episodes associated with penile pain and compulsive scratching of the carpet. He became fully dependent for all activities of daily living, including dressing, bathing, and feeding and became wheelchair-bound. At his last cognitive screen he could not even begin the trail-test or cube-copying tasks as part of the MoCA screen and dropped his MMSE score to 10/28, indicating severe generalized dementia. DLB was confirmed at autopsy.

Discussion: Although use of "atypical" neuroleptics may be regarded as safe in parkinsonian disorders, most of the drugs in this family can worsen motor features in PD and even the psychosis itself in DLB and the pathologically similar PD dementia. The physical and cognitive decline and increased mortality risk with the use of antipsychotics in DLB is referred to as "neuroleptic sensitivity," a core diagnostic feature. Supporting historical elements include fluctuations in cognition (and sometimes in consciousness), repeated falls, syncopal episodes, depression, delusions, and hallucinations. Even the typically "safe" neuroleptics, quetiapine and clozapine, may also cause symptomatic worsening.[25] Hence, careful monitoring of the use of neuroleptic agents is essential in DLB. The lower density of striatal dopamine D_2 receptors in DLB may account for both the limited response to levodopa and the increased sensitivity to neuroleptics.[26]

Cholinesterase inhibitors may be especially useful in the treatment of DLB, given the extent to which visual hallucinations, which are associated with impaired cognition and behavioral disturbances, are mediated by cholinergic deficits.[27] Importantly, neocortical cholinergic activity, particularly in the medial occipital cortex, is more severely depleted in DLB and PDD (with functionally intact post-synaptic muscarinic receptors) compared to AD.[28] Though promising, the antipsychotic efficacy of cholinergic drugs has not been formally studied in DLB or PDD.

Last three clinical pearls: First, among the synucleinopathies which RBD is believed to predate, DLB develops more commonly than PD or MSA, suggesting that premorbid RBD predicts greater severity of cognitive involvement, though apparently with less hallucinations and cognitive fluctuations compared to DLB patients without RBD.[24] Second, impairment of depth perception or impairment in "judging distance" and visuospatial disorientation localizes to the visual association areas in the bilateral occipitoparietal region (dorsal visual stream); involvement of this region suggests a diagnosis of DLB in the right clinical context (see also Case 43). And third, unlike AD, episodic memory (day-to-day events) is rarely affected early on in DLB patients. Conversely, AD patients rarely present with the impairments in visuospatial orientation which are typical in DLB.

Diagnosis: Neuroleptic sensitivity in dementia with Lewy bodies

Tip: *The psychosis and overall function of DLB worsen with all typical and most atypical antipsychotics. Clozapine is the most effective antipsychotic for patients in the PDD-DLB spectrum but quetiapine is a reasonable initial strategy.*

Case 53: When rigidity follows pain

Case: This 69-year-old man was admitted to the hospital for "inability to care for himself." He had a history of chronic pain due to multiple vertebral compression fractures and was on methadone 10 mg q.i.d and oxycodone/acetaminophen (5/325) as needed for breakthrough pain. He was also on citalopram 40 mg/day and trazodone 100 mg/day. At the hospital, his methadone was increased to 30 mg q.i.d. He complained of feeling restless and having leg cramps. On the third hospital day, his back pain worsened and methadone was increased again to 40 mg q.i.d. That evening, he became drowsy, only arousable to voice. His oxygen saturations were in the 80s and his breathing rate was only six times a minute. He was thought to have narcotic-induced hypoxia.

Would naloxone improve his restlessness and mental status changes?

Naloxone was tried but changed nothing. He was tachycardic in the 140s, hypertensive with a systolic blood pressure of 220 and with a temperature of 101.8°F. He vomited and was intubated due to inability to protect his airway. Rigidity and tremors were noted on admission to the MICU. While in the MICU he was placed on a fentanyl drip for 2 days along with continuing his methadone. Tachycardia, hypertension, and rigidity worsened while myoclonic movements appeared.

What is the revised diagnosis with the new data and failed naloxone trial?

At this point, the clinical diagnosis of serotonin syndrome (SS) can be safely made. This diagnosis prompted the removal of fentanyl and methadone from the regimen and the initiation of cyproheptadine, with 12 mg given initially, followed by 2 mg via nasogastric tube every 2 hours as needed, with a lorazepam drip. Off methadone and fentanyl and on cyproheptadine he slowly improved and was weaned off the supportive treatment 9 days later, and discharged home 2 weeks after that with no further sequelae.

Discussion: Methadone is a serotonin reuptake inhibitor which can induce serotonin toxicity alone or when combined with other SSRIs. In the absence of response to naloxone, the depressed sensorium as well as the autonomic and "neuromuscular" hyperactivity completed the picture of the serotonin syndrome.[29] The "neuromuscular" misnomer in the diagnostic triad actually refers to the central nervous system-generated myoclonus and leg-predominant rigidity, with or without accompanying tremor and hyperreflexia. Agitation, diaphoresis, and hyperpyrexia are often present, and may lead to diagnostic confusion with another neurological emergency associated with rigidity, the idiosyncratic neuroleptic malignant syndrome (NMS, Table 9.2). This overlap is hypothesized to relate to the impact that elevated serotonin levels have on lowering dopamine levels. Unlike NMS, patients with SS tend to have myoclonus, hyperreflexia, and restlessness.[30] The syndrome occurs with pharmacological increases in serotonin neurotransmission from excessive activation of 5-HT_{1A} and 5-HT_2 receptors through increased serotonin synthesis, decreased serotonin metabolism, increased serotonin release, inhibition of serotonin reuptake, or direct agonism of the serotonin receptors. A number of drugs with these mechanisms of action are capable of inducing SS, especially if combined (Table 9.3).

Table 9.2. Clinical and management differences between serotonin syndrome and neuroleptic malignant syndrome

Features	Serotonin syndrome	Neuroleptic malignant syndrome
Common to both	Encephalopathy, fever	Encephalopathy, fever
Dysautonomia	**Diarrhea**, excessive lacrimation, **mydriasis**	Hypertension, diaphoresis, incontinence
Rigidity	Leg-predominant rigidity	"Lead pipe" generalized rigidity
Tremor	Leg-predominant tremor	Full-body tremor
Myoclonus	**Present**, mostly in legs	Absent
Hyperreflexia	**Common**, mostly in legs	Rare

All distinguishing clinical features in serotonin syndrome are marked in bold. The other two neurological emergencies in the differential of serotonin syndrome are cholinergic toxicity (no rigidity, associated mydriasis) and malignant hyperthermia (hyporeflexia rather than hyperreflexia and "rigor mortis-like rigidity").

Table 9.3. Drugs causing serotonin syndrome

Inhibitors of serotonin reuptake	SSRIs, SNRIs, TCAs, dextromethorphan, dexamphetamine, cocaine, opiates (*excluding* morphine, codeine, oxycodone, and buprenorphine)
Inhibitors of serotonin metabolism	MAO-B inhibitors at high dose (selegiline), MAO-A inhibitors or non-selective MAOI antidepressants
Enhancers of serotonin synthesis	L-tryptophan, 5-HTP
Enhancers of serotonin release	MDMA (Ecstasy), amphetamines, cocaine, fenfluramine
Serotonin agonists	Sumatriptan and other triptans,* ergotamine, buspirone
Non-specific serotonin enhancers	Lithium, electroconvulsive therapy (ECT)

SSRIs, selective serotonin reuptake inhibitors; SNRIs, serotonin/norepinephrine reuptake inhibitors (venlafaxine, duloxetine); TCAs, tricyclic antidepressants; MAOIs, monoamine oxidase inhibitor.
* Triptans appear to be unlikely to cause full-blown serotonin syndrome by themselves or in combination with SSRIs.[34]
Adapted from Espay and Biller.[40]

Methadone is a synthetic phenylpiperidine opioid analgesic that acts as a μ opioid receptor agonist but also increases serotonin synthesis and inhibits its reuptake. Used in the management of chronic pain and maintenance of detoxification in opioid addiction, methadone has the potential to cause serotonin syndrome particularly when an SSRI antidepressant is part of the medication regimen.[31] Besides methadone, other synthetic phenylpiperidine opioids such as meperidine, tramadol, dextromethorphan and propoxyphene, also partly act as monoamine reuptake inhibitors and may induce SS when combined with MAO inhibitors.[32] Conversely, morphine, codeine, oxycodone and buprenorphine do not inhibit serotonin reuptake, and do not precipitate serotonin toxicity with MAOIs. The risk of SS is greatest, and its expression most severe, following the combination of any SSRI with an irreversible MAO-A or MAO-B inhibitor, even at therapeutic doses.[33] Conversely, overdose of these drugs in isolation may produce only mild serotonin toxicity. When pain control is urgent in critical care, anyone already on SSRIs, SNRIs, or TCAs should only be given the "safe" drugs morphine, codeine, oxycodone or buprenorphine, as most other opioids, particularly meperidine, can induce SS when added to a regimen with the above drugs. Treatment consists of discontinuation of the causative agent, supportive therapy, and cyproheptadine hydrochloride, an antihistamine and 5-HT$_{2A}$ antagonist, or chlorpromazine, a 5-HT$_{1A}$ and 5-HT$_2$ antagonist neuroleptic, for severe cases.

Diagnosis: Serotonin syndrome

Case 54: Poor response to L-dopa, poor response to DBS

Contributed by Drs. Shawn Smyth, Joseph Savitt, Stephen Grill, and Zoltan Mari, Johns Hopkins University, Baltimore, Maryland

Case: This 47-year-old woman with a history of depression, cervical spine disease, and restless legs syndrome developed progressive left-sided clumsiness, rest and kinetic hand tremor, bradykinesia, and rigidity. By 2 years into her symptoms, she had hypophonia, hypomimia, micrographia, constipation, left-hand dystonia, and slowed gait. A diagnosis of PD was made. Treatment with amantadine caused throat tightening and pramipexole, excessive fatigue, and lower extremity edema. By 3 to 4 years, she had developed urinary frequency, monotone hypophonia, mild dysphagia, sialorrhea, and presumed REM sleep behavior disorder. L-dopa provided excellent benefits in coordination, tremor, dystonia and hypophonia, but only minimally improved balance and gait. Motor complications emerged in the form of dyskinesias and left hand and foot "off" dystonia. By 5 years, she showed slight hypermetric saccades, dysarthria, and a cautious and unsteady gait, with tandem impairment, requiring a walker for ambulation. STN DBS implantation was offered after confirming sufficient response to L-dopa as measured by the UPDRS motor score improving from 25 in the "off" state to 17 in the "on" medication state (Video 54).

What elements of the history and exam rendered her a poor candidate for DBS?

The relatively rapid accrual of deficits should have been of concern, particularly her tandem gait impairment and the need for a walker within 5 years from symptom onset. Other red flags included oculomotor impairment, dysarthria, and dysphagia.

The overall benefit from STN DBS was mild, better for rigidity than bradykinesia, but limited by voltage-dependent stimulation-induced dyskinesias on each side, contralateral to the stimulated STN. A careful review of her brain MRI demonstrated a pattern of pontocerebellar atrophy not previously recognized (Figure 9.5).

In view of her progression and neuroimaging abnormalities, her diagnosis was revised to probable MSA. She went on to develop bilateral foot dystonia, fatigue with chewing, frequent trunk and limb dyskinesias, worsened sialorrhea, weakened cough, orthostatic hypotension, and urinary incontinence. She remained on frequent dosing of levodopa, entacapone, and bromocriptine as well as botulinum toxin injections for limb dystonia, with modest symptomatic benefit. Death occurred during the eighth year of illness due to aspiration pneumonia and subsequent medical complications. Brain autopsy confirmed MSA, showing atrophy and neuronal loss in the substantia nigra, pons, and inferior olive, and glial cytoplasmic inclusions in the medulla, inferior olive, pons, midbrain, cerebellum, cingulate, and neocortex. The lack of striatal involvement is consistent with the "minimal change" variant of MSA, where cell loss and glial inclusions remain mainly confined to the pigmented brain stem nuclei and cerebellum.[35] As in this patient, severe L-dopa induced dyskinesias have been reported as a feature of this form of MSA.[36]

Discussion: Several lessons were drawn from this case. The first, and perhaps the most important, is that rapid accrual of deficits, reaching an early walker-dependent motor milestone, is a major red flag against the diagnosis of PD. The second is that, although the absolute reduction of motor deficits may have met a pre-defined definition of L-dopa "responsiveness," the patient's relative residual disability remained substantial after achieving L-dopa peak-dose benefits during the off-on dose study. This was particularly the case for gait and balance, which are least improved by surgical treatments. And, finally, this case highlights the perils of considering early STN DBS for patients with PD-like

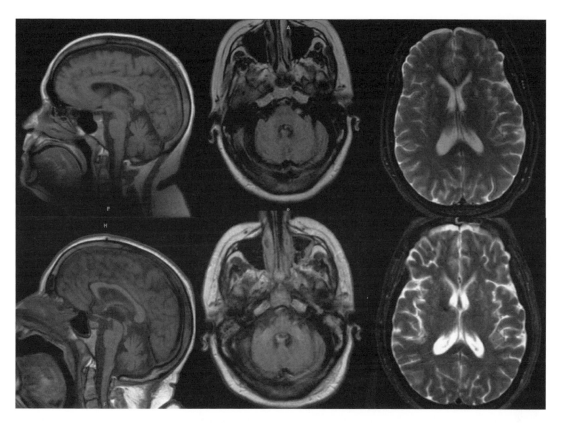

Figure 9.5. T1-weighted, FLAIR, and T2-weighted brain MRI 4 years (upper row) and 6 years (lower row, after STN DBS implantation) after disease onset. Notice interval atrophy of the pons and cerebellar vermis, with increased abnormal signal in the middle cerebellar peduncle and, to a lesser extent, in the putaminal region.

disorders, treated at a time when overt signs of an alternative diagnosis may not yet have become apparent. In these cases, the outcome will be invariably poor, with any early benefit rapidly vanishing.

MSA is arguably the most common asymmetric akinetic-rigid syndrome that mimics PD, including a potentially robust early response to L-dopa compared to all other "unresponsive or poorly L-dopa-responsive" atypical parkinsonisms.[37;38] Indeed, this patient's L-dopa response, which included asymmetric limb dyskinesias, was of a magnitude that falsely reassured her neurologist of a diagnosis of PD and prompted consideration of surgical treatment.[39] The features that supported MSA, including orthostatic hypotension and urinary

dysfunction, did not occur until later in the disease. Earlier development of hypermetric saccades and tandem impairment were neglected given the appearance of "typical" PD dyskinesias and a relatively sustained, if imperfect, response to L-dopa.

Diagnosis: Multiple system atrophy, "minimal change" variant.

Tip: *DBS should not be considered when disability becomes severe within five years from onset of "PD" symptoms. Diagnoses other than PD are common among those who reach a walker- or wheelchair-dependent state within such time frame, reducing the long-term benefits of DBS and sometimes hastening disease progression.*

REFERENCES

1. Pahwa R, Factor SA, Lyons KE, et al. Practice Parameter: treatment of Parkinson disease with motor fluctuations and dyskinesia (an evidence-based review): report of the Quality Standards Subcommittee of the American Academy of Neurology. *Neurology* 2006;**66**(7):983–995.

2. Silver DE, Sahs AL. Livedo reticularis in Parkinson's disease patients treated with amantadine hydrochloride. *Neurology* 1972;**22**(7):665–669.

3. Wolf E, Seppi K, Katzenschlager R, et al. Long-term antidyskinetic efficacy of amantadine in Parkinson's disease. *Mov Disord* 2010;**25**(10):1357–1363.

4. Poewe W. When a Parkinson's disease patient starts to hallucinate. *Pract Neurol* 2008;**8**(4):238–241.

5. Lang AE. When and how should treatment be started in Parkinson disease? *Neurology* 2009;**72** (7 Suppl):S39–S43.

6. Fernandez HH, Friedman JH. Classification and treatment of tardive syndromes. *Neurologist* 2003;**9** (1):16–27.

7. Casey DE, Denney D. Pharmacological characterization of tardive dyskinesia. *Psychopharmacology (Berl)* 1977;**54**(1):1–8.

8. Bai YM, Yu SC, Lin CC. Risperidone for severe tardive dyskinesia: a 12-week randomized, double-blind, placebo-controlled study. *J Clin Psychiatry* 2003;**64** (11):1342–1348.

9. Dalack GW, Becks L, Meador-Woodruff JH. Tardive dyskinesia, clozapine, and treatment response. *Prog Neuropsychopharmacol Biol Psychiatry* 1998;**22** (4):567–573.

10. Aia PG, Revuelta GJ, Cloud LJ, et al. Tardive dyskinesia. *Curr Treat Options Neurol* 2011;**13** (3):231–241.

11. Tarsy D, Baldessarini RJ. Epidemiology of tardive dyskinesia: is risk declining with modern antipsychotics? *Mov Disord* 2006;**21**(5):589–598.

12. Quinn N. The "round the houses" sign in progressive supranuclear palsy. *Ann Neurol* 1996;**40**(6):951.

13. Morariu MA. Progressive supranuclear palsy and normal-pressure hydrocephalus. *Neurology* 1979;**29** (11):1544–1546.

14. Curran T, Lang AE. Parkinsonian syndromes associated with hydrocephalus: case reports, a review of the literature, and pathophysiological hypotheses. *Mov Disord* 1994;**9**(5):508–520.

15. Hamilton R, Patel S, Lee EB, et al. Lack of shunt response in suspected idiopathic normal pressure hydrocephalus with Alzheimer disease pathology. *Ann Neurol* 2010;**68**(4):535–540.

16. Ananth J, Edelmuth E, Dargan B. Meige's syndrome associated with neuroleptic treatment. *Am J Psychiatry* 1988;**145**(4):513–515.

17. Kanovsky P, Streitova H, Bares M, et al. Treatment of facial and orolinguomandibular tardive dystonia by botulinum toxin A: evidence of a long-lasting effect. *Mov Disord* 1999;**14**(5):886–888.

18. Reese R, Gruber D, Schoenecker T, et al. Long-term clinical outcome in Meige syndrome treated with internal pallidum deep brain stimulation. *Mov Disord* 2011;**26**(4):691–698.

19. LeDoux MS. Meige syndrome: what's in a name? *Parkinsonism Relat Disord* 2009;**15**(7):483–489.

20. Weintraub D, Koester J, Potenza MN, et al. Impulse control disorders in Parkinson disease: a cross-sectional study of 3090 patients. *Arch Neurol* 2010;**67** (5):589–595.

21. Weintraub D, Sohr M, Potenza MN, et al. Amantadine use associated with impulse control disorders in Parkinson disease in cross-sectional study. *Ann Neurol* 2010;**68**(6):963–968.

22. O'Sullivan SS, Evans AH, Lees AJ. Dopamine dysregulation syndrome: an overview of its epidemiology, mechanisms and management. *CNS Drugs* 2009;**23** (2):157–170.

23. Ahlskog JE. Pathological behaviors provoked by dopamine agonist therapy of Parkinson's disease. *Physiol Behav* 2011;**104**(1):168–172.

24. Postuma RB, Gagnon JF, Vendette M, et al. Idiopathic REM sleep behavior disorder in the transition to degenerative disease. *Mov Disord* 2009;**24**(15):2225–2232.

25. Kobayashi A, Kawanishi C, Matsumura T, et al. Quetiapine-induced neuroleptic malignant syndrome in dementia with Lewy bodies: a case report. *Prog Neuropsychopharmacol Biol Psychiatry* 2006;**30** (6):1170–1172.

26. Piggott MA, Marshall EF, Thomas N, et al. Striatal dopaminergic markers in dementia with Lewy bodies, Alzheimer's and Parkinson's diseases: rostrocaudal distribution. *Brain* 1999;**122** (Pt 8):1449–1468.

27. Henriksen AL, St Dennis C, Setter SM, et al. Dementia with Lewy bodies: therapeutic opportunities and pitfalls. *Consult Pharm* 2006;**21**(7):563–575.

28. Benarroch EE. Acetylcholine in the cerebral cortex: effects and clinical implications. *Neurology* 2010;**75** (7):659–665.

29. Boyer EW, Shannon M. The serotonin syndrome. *N Engl J Med* 2005;**352**(11):1112–1120.

30. Robottom BJ, Weiner WJ, Factor SA. Movement disorders emergencies part 1: hypokinetic disorders. *Arch Neurol* 2011;**68**(5):567–572.

31. Martinez TT, Martinez DN. A case of serotonin syndrome associated with methadone overdose. *Proc West Pharmacol Soc* 2008;**51**:42–44.

32. Gillman PK. Monoamine oxidase inhibitors, opioid analgesics and serotonin toxicity. *Br J Anaesth* 2005;**95**(4):434–441.

33. Gillman PK. A review of serotonin toxicity data: implications for the mechanisms of antidepressant drug action. *Biol Psychiatry* 2006;**59** (11):1046–1051.

34. Gillman K. Serotonin toxicity. *Headache* 2008;**48** (4):640–641.

35. Wenning GK, Quinn N, Magalhaes M, et al. "Minimal change" multiple system atrophy. *Mov Disord* 1994;**9** (2):161–166.

36. Huang Y, Garrick R, Cook R, et al. Pallidal stimulation reduces treatment-induced dyskinesias in "minimal-change" multiple system atrophy. *Mov Disord* 2005;**20** (8):1042–1047.

37. Constantinescu R, Richard I, Kurlan R. Levodopa responsiveness in disorders with parkinsonism: a review of the literature. *Mov Disord* 2007;**22**(15):2141–2148.

38. Hughes AJ, Daniel SE, Kilford L, et al. Accuracy of clinical diagnosis of idiopathic Parkinson's disease: a clinico-pathological study of 100 cases. *J Neurol Neurosurg Psychiatry* 1992;**55**(3):181–184.

39. Shih LC, Tarsy D. Deep brain stimulation for the treatment of atypical parkinsonism. *Mov Disord* 2007;**22** (15):2149–2155.

40. Espay AJ, Biller J. *Concise Neurology.* Philadelphia, PA: Lippincott Williams & Wilkins, division of Wolters Kluwer Health, Inc., 2011.

Appendix: Video Legends

Case 1: Upbeat nystagmus and wide-based gait are shown in a patient shortly discharged from the psychiatric ward for acute personality changes and memory deficits.

Case 2a: Gait is wide based, toes are externally rotated, arm swinging is normal relative to the slow gait, and posture shows little to no stooping. These features have been typically described in vascular parkinsonism.

Case 2b: Gait shows a marked improvement (> 40% in gait velocity) after a 3-day external lumbar drainage in-hospital procedure.

Case 2c: A patient with PD demonstrated festination with freeezing compared to the patient described here, in which festination did not manifest despite our asking the patient to hasten his gait.

Case 3a: Examination emphasizes the discrepancy between a marked reduction in the cervical range of motion due to axial rigidity with restoration of the full mobility upon voluntary movements. Overlooked features in this assessment include the asymmetric decrement in the amplitude of finger tapping and ipsilateral reduction in arm swinging, which would have steered the diagnosis in the right direction.

Case 3b: Same patient after 100 mg thrice daily of L-dopa, showing improvement of hypokinetic and rigid features and normalization of the arm swinging during walking.

Case 3c: Two examples of disorders demonstrating hypokinesia but not typically considered within the realm of parkinsonisms: stiff-person syndrome (as suspected in the patient previously discussed) and primary lateral sclerosis (video case courtesy of Dr. Héctor González Usigli, Instituto Mexicano del Seguro Social, Guadalajara, Jalisco, México).

Case 4a: Left hemifacial myoclonic movements are shown at examination, approximately 6 months after symptom onset. Note the disappearance of the movements during voluntary tasks (grimacing, tongue protrusion, etc).

Case 4b: Almost no abnormal movements are documented during his examination 2 months after initiation of treatment with carbamazepine, after reaching dose of 1400 mg/day.

Case 5: 66-year-old diabetic seamstress demonstrating episodes of intermittent painful hand posturing, typical of tetany. Five-minute episodes of sudden-onset of left thumb adduction and index finger extension are reported as painful.

Case 6a: Tremor of the right hand that is apparent on rest and posture but disappears with passive manipulation of the contralateral arm. There is intermittent right foot tremor but no entrainment or disappearance with passive and voluntary tasks of other limbs (video case courtesy of Dr. Francesca Morgante, Università di Messina, Sicily, Italy).

Case 6b: Foot tremor is sustained only when the anterior aspect of the sole is supported (which allows the use of physiologic clonus) and disappears when the entire sole of the foot lies flat against the ground (when physiologic clonus is impossible). Other features shown for this tremor include variability of amplitude, frequency, and distribution (migration of tremor proximally in the leg when testing resistance), as well as the accompanying give-way weakness.

Case 7a: Mild left toe elevation during walking. He imitated a kicking movement of the left leg expected to occur with longer walking.

Case 7b: Highlighted examination features include generalized hyperreflexia, with absent jaw jerk but prominent leg spasticity, ankle clonus, and Babinski reflexes. These were unexpected findings for "pure" stiff-person syndrome. Notice that the muscle tone testing of the left leg includes a spastic catch from spasticity and a slow relaxation phase from concurrent rigidity.

Case 8a: Rest and postural hand myoclonus are seen. Once standing, she reported "weakness" and unsteadiness, which worsened the longer she remained erect. With the naked eye, it would have been nearly impossible to discern that the abnormal movements in her legs were myoclonic (as revealed later by electrophysiology). She experienced relief when walking, which was slow and cautious.

Case 8b: A classic phenotype of advanced orthostatic tremor, with rapid elicitation and worsening of unsteadiness upon standing with more visible jerking, which could have been suspected as myoclonic (instead confirmed as a 16-Hz synchronous tremor on electrophysiology, diagnostic of orthostatic tremor). There was substantial relief of symptoms upon walking. The longer she walked the better her gait became.

Case 9: Slowed and hypophonic dysarthric speech ("hypo/bradyphonia"), pseudobulbar affect with inappropriate laughter, supranuclear vertical gaze paresis, weakness of orbicularis oculi, proximal leg weakness, and gait and balance impairment.

Case 10a: Patient description of her symptoms in the right facial region. The abnormality is best palpated than seen.

Case 10b: EMG of the right temporalis and right masseter of the same patient showed spontaneous recurring discharges, both monosynaptic and polysynaptic. Polysynaptic discharges had a frequency > 1 Hz but the monosynaptic discharges occurred at 20–30 Hz.

Case 11 contains no video.

Case 12: Truncal-greater-than-appendicular ataxia with hypokinetic movements that may be more dysmetric than parkinsonian.

Case 13a: Initial patient evaluation shows mild end-target kinetic tremor on the left hand with clearly asymmetric hypo- and bradykinesia on left hand and foot tapping. He also demonstrates how his previously proficient clog dancing has been affected by his left foot impairment. The last segment shows imperfect tandem gait, which further validates this simple task as a red flag, admittedly non-specific, against the diagnosis of PD.

Case 13b: The orofacial dyskinesia becomes evident during the interview; the patient initially remains unaware. The exam also discloses worsening of his hypokinetic movements, tandem gait, and postural reflexes.

Case 13c: A fully developed L-dopa-induced "risus sardonicus" in another patient with MSA. She demonstrates a sensory trick.

Case 13d: Three different patients with pathology-proven MSA demonstrating some atypical features ("red flags"): axial stimulus-sensitive myoclonus, orofacial dystonia, inconsistent or wide-based gait, postural impairment, orofacial dystonia with feet dyskinesias as L-dopa-induced complications, Pisa syndrome, and inspiratory stridor.

Case 14a: The "smirk" fragment of the "risus sardonicus" is present intermittently at rest and during speech in this patient with Wilson's disease.

Case 14b: Another patient with the characteristic "risus sardonicus" phenotype of facial dystonia due to Wilson's disease, associated with parkinsonism as shown by right-hand rest tremor, hypokinesia, and slowed gait (video case courtesy of Dr. Leo Verhagen).

Case 15a: Right-hand tremor, almost exclusively affecting the thumb, is shown first at "rest" (although perhaps with the arms insufficiently relaxed) enhanced during a mental task. Asymmetric flexion-extension tremor is of about similar magnitude in posture and action. Arm swinging was normal.

Case 15b: Marked anti-tremor benefit with propranolol, noted first 2 weeks after reaching 5 mg four times daily. Benefits have been sustained for six

years since this evaluation, albeit periodic dose increases have been required.

Case 15c: This patient first became aware of his right-hand tremor 6 years prior to this evaluation and progressively it interfered with feeding (spilling from a fork or spoon) and writing. Examination shows a resting, postural, and kinetic tremor whose latency to reappearance ("reemergence") is barely perceptible. Tremor is seen during handwriting – though notice the previously unapparent ipsilateral leg tremor. Right-hand tremor remains highly visible during walking.

Case 15d: Same patient as above, after introduction of L-dopa. The resting tremor has substantially attenuated, reappearing (as it does in the right leg) only when tapping the opposite hand. The postural component remains present.

Case 16a: This patient's "restlessness" is masked by a number of activities, but emerges more clearly as choreiform ("piano-playing") movements when holding the arms outstretched during a mental task. Writing does not cause exacerbation of movements or emergence of myoclonic jerks.

Case 16b: This patient's "restlessness" is subtle in the neck and trunk, but emerges more clearly as myoclonic movements when performing cognitive or motor tasks, such as drinking or, most especially, writing. At the end of the segment, his brother's predominantly axial myoclonic jerks are shown while writing (video case courtesy of Dr. Cindy Zadikoff, Northwestern University's Feinberg School of Medicine, Chicago, IL).

Case 17a: This patient demonstrates mild postural tremor, hypokinesia, and a subtle orofacial dyskinesia about which he is unaware.

Case 17b: This 58-year-old man demonstrates the classic "rabbit tremor" of drug-induced parkinsonism. He was treated with valproate and risperidone for chronic paranoid schizophrenia. Sequential tapering of both of these drugs markedly improved this feature, his hand tremor, and his gait, without psychiatric decompensation.

Case 18a: The patient has difficulty with relating her problems, with frequent speech arrests. There are subtle myoclonic movements in the orofacial region and her hands, when the arms are held outstretched.

Case 18b: Reduction in the dose of amantadine restores her speech and eliminates the subtle myoclonic orofacial and hand movements.

Case 19: The rapid alternating movements may be slightly hypokinetic but exhibit no decrement or fatiguing. The hands showed subtle finger posturing and arrhythmic jerking when the arms were held outstretched. Handwriting is not micrographic. Next segment, 2 years later (still without treatment): Examination showed end-target jerky tremor without dysmetria. Arm swinging remains preserved.

Case 20a: The patient describes episodes of left arm levitation and exhibits high-frequency, high-amplitude unilateral tremor on his most affected, dystonic arm. His gait is hemiparetic, further highlighting the markedly asymmetric phenotype.

Case 20b: Case of CBS with pathology-proven AD in a 79-year-old with a 7-year course of markedly asymmetric parkinsonism with aphasia. At onset, his family noticed frequent "jerks" of his left arm and leg. His balance worsened and he would tend to lean to the left; he would "stall" with freezing of gait. He had trouble figuring out how to sit down on a toilet seat and needed assistance with dressing, grooming, eating. His left hand would sometimes "wander" and go into his pocket or grab his shirt, without his knowledge. He showed no response to L-dopa. Exam at 3 years from onset demonstrated aphasia, severe ideomotor apraxia, left greater than right, left arm dystonia, intermittent myoclonus, left greater than right, and a Babinski response extensor bilaterally (video case courtesy of Dr. Andrew Duker, University of Cincinnati, Cincinnati, OH).

Case 21: The patient demonstrated postural and kinetic tremor of relatively high frequency but low amplitude. Arm swinging was normal. His drug list is shown at the end, in the patient's own finely jagged handwriting.

Case 22a: Difficult to characterize movements, during the initial evaluation. Though the movements may have been interpreted as "tremulous," they were arrhythmic, of varying but overall small amplitude, and were not influenced by positional changes. Individual fingers seemed to move asynchronously and had a jerky component, slower than expected for myoclonus. There was no clear posturing of the fingers.

Case 22b: The patient is examined after an episode of pain and swelling in the knees and finger joints. The movements seem less prominent compared with the finger edema. Last segment demonstrates that pain and swelling have been controlled with prednisone. Residual movements are also attenuated. Facial myokymia has newly appeared.

Case 23: Patient admitted to being clumsy and "tipsy". The examination shows occasional jerks in the face. Some neck and truncal swaying may represent axial ataxia but intermixed chorea was possible. Ocular examination shows oculomotor apraxia and intermittent large-amplitude saccadic intrusions. There were some myoclonic jerks in the face and right limbs, which were correlated with epileptic EEG activity.

Case 24a: Patient demonstrates spastic dysarthria. Rapid alternating movements of hands and feet are slow and hypokinetic but there is no decrement or fatiguing. Gait is slow and spastic. Postural reflexes are impaired. Hyperreflexia with Babinski is shown (video case courtesy of Dr. Héctor González Usigli, Instituto Mexicano del Seguro Social, Guadalajara, Jalisco, México).

Case 24b: Gait of a patient with anti-GAD-positive stiff-person syndrome. The excessive parkinsonian-like slowness is contributed to by her fear of falling, a common complaint in these patients (despite a truly rare rate of falls).

Case 25 contains no video.

Case 26: This young woman displays a state of "wakeful unresponsiveness" in the setting of choreiform movements of the face and random but conjugate saccadic movements.

Case 27a: This 31-year-old man shows mild tongue protrusion with feeding and lower face dystonic movements. Low chorein level confirmed chorea-acanthocytosis (ChAc) (video case courtesy of Dr. Ruth Walker, Mount Sinai School of Medicine and the James J. Peters Veterans Affairs Medical Center in the Bronx, New York).

Case 27b: This 82-year-old woman also exhibits generalized chorea with predominant involvement of the orofacial region, affecting chewing, for over 30 years. There was no true tongue protrusion at rest or during chewing, documented at the end of the video segment. Despite a history suggestive of feeding dystonia, reminiscent of the prior case (27a), her chewing was relatively spared. The long history of exposure to risperidone, her late age of onset (mean age of onset in ChAc is around 30), and her lack of true progression or weight loss distinguished this case of tardive dyskinesia from ChAc. Also, there was no increased CK and the chorein assay was normal.

Case 28 contains no video.

Case 29a: Severe painful oromandibular dystonia and blepharospasm, present at rest but exacerbated during speech. There is dystonia of the hands and fingers noted on arms outstretched and during walking.

Case 29b: Within 20 minutes from an intervention (see text) improvement of his dystonia at rest was appreciated with resolution of blepharospasm and reduction in pain. Still significant speech-induced dystonia of the oromandibular region remained, though it continued to improve over the subsequent 3 weeks.

Case 30a: Postural and kinetic tremor of the hands, with involvement of her voice. The tremor increases with weight as shown during strength testing. Her gait showed normal arm swing without tremor but some impairment of tandem and postural reflexes.

Case 30b: On re-examination, 2 years later, she had a jerkier element to her hand tremor and a previously unrecognized head tremor. She demonstrates that changes in position of the arm alter the magnitude of the tremor.

Case 30c: This 76-year-old man has had slowly progressive asymmetric tremor for 4 years, more prominent in the left hand. He is most concerned about his handwriting, which is jerky but not small.

Case 30d: Same patient as above after reaching a dose of 300 mg/day of primidone. Notice the marked improvement in the tremor and the finger tapping task, and moderate improvement in spiral drawing. Interestingly, he acknowledges an element of position specificity when the tremor increases as he draws the spiral.

Case 31a: Semi-rhythmic contractions of the mid- and lower face, including jaw-closing muscles and platysma, associated with convergent-divergent oscillations and intermittent left blepharospasm. Note his impaired horizontal pursuit and complete inability to initiate vertical gaze. These deficits are overcome by oculocephalic maneuvers (not shown).

Case 31b: Similar myorhythmia without the convergent-divergent oscillations but with clear horizontal and vertical supranuclear gaze palsy (video courtesy of Dr. Catherine Zahn, Toronto Western Hospital, Toronto, ON).

Case 32: Generalized dyskinesias with prominent ballistic component of the legs. Notice the marked improvement following a subcutaneous injection with apomorphine (video case courtesy of Dr. Leo Verhagen, Rush-Presbyterian, Chicago, IL).

Case 33: Progressively worsening eversion and plantar flexion of the right foot which persists after the end of brisk walking on treadmill.

Case 34 contains no video.

Case 35: Notice the variability from jerk to jerk, and the effects on them by finger tapping and wrist rotation tasks. Additional effects on timing (entrainment) and direction of the head movements are shown (video case courtesy of Dr. Don Gilbert, Cincinnati Children's Hospital, University of Cincinnati, Cincinnati, OH).

Case 36: The first segment shows patient at age 14 years, before the introduction of L-dopa, with hypophonic and labored voice and hypokinetic movements. Some dystonic facial movements can be seen. In the second segment, at age 17, she is on L-dopa and displays dystonic and choreoathetotic movements in her face, tongue, and hands (first video segment courtesy of Dr. Leo Verhagen, Rush-Presbyterian, Chicago, IL).

Case 37: Video segments demonstrated hypermetric saccades, ankle dorsiflexor weakness, dysmetria on finger-to-nose and, to a greater extent, heel-to-shin. Heel-to-shin task performance using her right leg was limited by substantial weakness. Her gait showed a waddle component and wide base. She could not stand on her feet without support.

Case 38: Patient describes her symptoms while in her "off" state. Non-motor symptoms in the form of anxiety predominate. Although the patient showed intermittent left-hand tremor, she is most concerned about the pain in the same arm and the anxiety and inattention that develop when L-dopa wears off. Finger-to-nose testing showed mild dystonic tremor. Fatigability of left-hand finger tapping and decreased arm swing revealed her parkinsonism despite a largely hyperkinetic flavor to her clinical picture given by her anxious demeanor.

Case 39: Hyperkinetic movements in the form of chorea and tics are seen both during action and at rest. The movements affect predominantly the face during rest and hands during posture. She demonstrates the partially suppressible throat clearing. Her gait shows some swaying with variable base of support and retropulsion on pull test.

Case 40: As the interview reveals details of her prior episodes, a variably oscillatory behavior is seen that falls between tremor and chorea. Although one can see how the diagnosis of chorea may have been considered in the past, tremor is the predominant phenotype. The tremor in both hands is variable. There are also intermittent platysma contractions with pulling of the lower lips, synchronous with the semi-rhythmic axial activity. Her speech shows typical psychogenic stuttering. At the end of the video, the patient's tremor disappeared or substantially changed in appearance and frequency and during distracting maneuvers.

Case 41a: Examination showed moderate akinesia with left-hand dystonia and tremor, the latter more pronounced during finger-to-nose task and on gait. There was decreased arm swinging on the left and mildly impaired tandem gait with preserved postural reflexes.

Case 41b: Examination on follow-up of the same patient, after reaching a dose of 150 mg three times daily of L-dopa, demonstrated marked improvement in her parkinsonism but development of leg dyskinesias and lower face dystonia, more prominently after each dose of L-dopa.

Case 42: Video shows high-amplitude, low-frequency postural and action tremor predominantly of the upper limbs and mild truncal ataxia, which is magnified during the tandem gait task (patient was wearing a mask during the 2003 SARS epidemic).

Case 43a: Oculomotor examination showed fragments of optic ataxia, an impairment of visual navigation expressed as her inability to accurately follow a target. Her severe dementia reduces the magnitude of this highly localizing sign (unlike a better developed manifestation in the next case). She shows prominent parkinsonism and clear postural impairment, far beyond what would have been expected of PD within 5 years from onset of symptoms.

Case 43b: 71-year-old man with parkinsonism, dementia, and prominent hallucinations, with probable dementia with Lewy bodies, demonstrating full Balint syndrome due to a posterior-predominant cortical pattern of atrophy. Optic ataxia and simultanagnosia are prominent. Ocular apraxia is not shown.

Case 44a: Asymmetric performance of finger tapping and left ideomotor apraxia to a transitive gesture is shown. The patient tends to lean sideways. Although stride length does not seem compromised when using a walker and her base is not wide, she is markedly posturally impaired and at great risk for falls. There was no true freezing or motor block but more overt right-sided swaying when crossing the doorway.

Case 44b: This segment demonstrates square-wave jerks, saccadic pursuit on right gaze, and hypometric saccades in the same patient. There was mild dysmetria and dysdiadochokinesia on the right hand.

Case 45: Marked resting and, to a lesser extent, postural tremor. Decrement with finger tapping indicates true bradykinesia (video segment courtesy of Dr. Leo Verhagen, Rush-Presbyterian, Chicago, IL).

Case 46: Dysarthria, cervical and oro-buccal dyskinesias, with frontalis overactivation and dystonic posturing of neck and left upper limb are shown (video segment courtesy of Dr. Alex Lehn, Princess Alexandra Hospital, Brisbane, QLD, Australia).

Case 47a: Severely disabled parkinsonian man exhibiting spontaneous resting and postural myoclonic movements in the hands and neck, intermittent right-hand tremor, marked postural and gait impairments. He could barely take a few steps. Livedo reticularis is also shown in the thighs.

Case 47b: The same patient 2 months after the elimination of amantadine, reduction of pramipexole, and increase in L-dopa/carbidopa/entacapone, showing no residual tremor and restoration of gait. Postural myoclonus is markedly reduced and livedo reticularis no longer apparent.

Case 48a: Orolingual movements in a patient with prior exposure to aripiprazole. Note that there is no interference with speech and no tongue protrusion impersistence. There is mild dystonic posturing at the fingers and end-target tremor, with fatiguing of rapid alternating movements. There is a slow, cautious gait, and impaired postural reflexes.

Case 48b: Movements are much improved after discontinuation of benztropine. Residual hand tremor is minimal.

Case 48c: Patient has the classical manifestations of tardive dystonia: paroxysmal retrocollis and arching backwards of the trunk, internal rotation of the arms, extension at the elbows, and flexion at the wrists.

Case 49a: The video shows impaired optokinetic oculomotor response and errors in performance of transitive gestures, which may represent limb kinetic apraxia. Movements are clumsy but not clearly bradykinetic. Gait is wide based and postural reflexes are impaired.

Case 49b: The video shows widening of gait and impairment of balance. The impairment of upgaze with slowed vertical saccades and the "round the houses" sign are demonstrated.

Case 50a: Dystonic contractions of cranial muscles are shown, causing intermittent tongue protrusion and jaw opening dystonia that interfered with speech.

Case 50b: Same case demonstrating improvement with tetrabenazine 75 mg daily, but with the clear development of masking of his face.

Case 50c: Tongue tremor, braykinesia and more marked masked facies developed at a dose of tetrabenazine of 125 mg daily.

Case 50d: Rebound worsening of the cranial dystonia, with more pronounced jaw opening and tongue involvement, is appreciated after discontinuation of tetrabenazine.

Case 51 contains no video.

Case 52: An episode of erratic behaviors ("wanted to rip his face") with shouting and gesturing reported in this home video made by his spouse. She indicated that he had been fluctuating between normal behavior and shouting, with increasing hallucinations.

Case 53 contains no video.

Case 54: The video demonstrates the off-on behaviour on this patient, as part of her consideration for STN DNS implantation 6 years after symptom onset of presumed PD. L-dopa yielded moderate improvements in hypokinesia and gait impairment (video courtesy of Dr. Shawn Smyth, Johns Hopkins University, Baltimore, Maryland).

Index

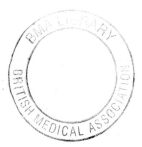